WHY
YOU
CAN'T
GO

Lorraine Cooney is a specialist gastroenterology dietitian at Dublin's Blackrock Clinic, where she leads the Gut Health Clinic. She specialises in managing conditions such as constipation and irritable bowel syndrome (IBS). Her passion fuels her mission: to empower people to gain back control of their digestive well-being and break free from the anxiety and the burden that often accompany gut problems.

Lorraine is a co-author of the popular low FODMAP recipe book and reference guide *Gut Feeling*, a guest lecturer on digestive conditions, and proudly chairs the award-winning Gastro Dietitians Interest Group in Ireland.

WHY YOU CAN'T GO

... and what you can do
to find life-changing relief
from constipation

Lorraine Cooney

Registered Dietitian

Gill Books

Gill Books
Hume Avenue
Park West
Dublin 12
www.gillbooks.ie

Gill Books is an imprint of M.H. Gill and Co.

978 1 8045 8046 2

Edited by Gráinne Treanor
Indexed by Eileen O'Neill
Printed and bound in Great Britain by
    Clays Ltd, Elcograf S.p.A.
Design and print origination by iota
    (www.iota-books.ie)
Illustrations by Lydia Moran
This book is typeset in Minion and
    Brandon Grotesque.

*The paper used in this book comes from the
wood pulp of sustainably managed forests.*

This book is not intended as a substitute for
the medical advice of a health professional.

A CIP catalogue record for this book is
available from the British Library.

5 4 3 2 1

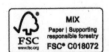

CONTENTS

A MESSAGE FROM THE AUTHOR

The intricacies of the human gut, much like the rest of the body, hold vast mysteries yet to be unravelled. To understand conditions such as constipation and their wide-ranging impacts – and to go beyond cultural traditions, old wives' tales and contemporary non-medical trendsetters – we rely on science. Science itself, however, is not always black and white. And it's always dynamic and evolving –a method or process of understanding and discovery.

In this book, you'll find valuable insights and recommendations that come from a thorough examination of trustworthy research papers and learnings I have gained from my dietetic colleagues; gastroenterologists, general practitioners and pelvic health physiotherapists; as well as conferences and courses. You'll also find practical wisdom acquired over several decades of hands-on clinical experience. It's important that you receive the most current and best-informed advice available.

When reading this book, you'll also discover many instances where strong evidence for certain practices or recommendations is not always available. However, this absence of robust scientific backing does not necessarily imply ineffectiveness. Having direct contact with patients and guiding them in addressing their constipation issues is invaluable for knowing what to advise. Its significance goes beyond anecdotal evidence where extensive scientific research is limited. The aim of this book is to embody this balanced perspective, promoting a method to manage constipation that is both scientifically informed and rooted in practical clinical experience. The hope is that it benefits those who suffer with this stubborn problem without any undue harm.

As you delve into this book, you'll also come to realise that constipation management isn't always straightforward. At times, it's even compared to an art form! The aim is to empower you with a deep understanding of all the ins and outs of constipation and help you identify changes that can enhance your sense of control. This will position you to achieve constipation relief and lead to a considerable improvement in your well-being.

Why did I write a book on constipation?

In my Gut Health Clinic at the Blackrock Clinic in Dublin, I've met countless individuals, all adults, struggling with constipation. In fact, constipation stands out as the most common and persistent issue among my patients. It includes not only chronic constipation but also cases of irritable bowel syndrome predominant constipation or IBS-C. I've noticed that so many people really don't get the opportunity to understand what constipation is all about, or how to handle it. And that's exactly why I was motivated to write this book.

Every page in this book will provide you with a wealth of knowledge and practical insights to help you understand constipation, along with what genuinely works and what might work (there are lots of these!) – and caution against what doesn't. Whether you're seeking answers to common questions or exploring effective strategies for relief, this book is your trusted companion on your journey to better digestive health.

While the book can serve as a comprehensive guide, it's essential to remember it's for educational purposes only, and for people over 18 years of age. If you're battling the dreaded constipation, it is best to use this resource in conjunction with your healthcare team. To make your life easier, it's best to have these in your corner: your doctor and/or gastroenterologist, a gut health dietitian and a pelvic health physiotherapist to help you join the dots and smooth out your path for a constipation-free existence.

The structure of the book

Chapter 1 introduces constipation and discusses the stigma and taboos surrounding the condition, as well as historical treatments.

Chapter 2 delves into the digestive system, because understanding what's going on with constipation is much easier when we understand how our digestive system works. It includes a candid conversation about 'poo'!

Chapter 3 looks in more detail at what is happening when we experience constipation. It includes statistics for constipation; the diagnosis of the condition and what we can expect during a visit to the doctor; red flags; types of constipation; causes of and risk factors for constipation; and consequences of the condition, including the impact on quality of life.

In Chapter 4 we step into the fascinating world of our gut microbiome, where trillions of tiny inhabitants play a vital role in our health.

Chapter 5 gives you an opportunity to get personal, profiling your own constipation by categorising your poo, exploring your current food choices and lifestyle, and tracking your habits – helping you piece together your experience of constipation.

In Chapters 6, 7 and 8 you'll find the low-down on the evidence base for choosing foods that will help relieve and prevent constipation. Chapter 6 explains the role of diet and especially fibre; Chapter 7 explores fibre foods, providing a useful directory; and Chapter 8 delves into fibre supplements, continuing the fibre directory begun in Chapter 7.

Chapter 9 looks at what else might be lurking behind a person's response to diet. It explores side effects of fibre, what to do if fibre is not working, how to increase fibre intake, and the bothersome issue of fibre anxiety. We look beyond fibre in Chapter 10 to the role of other foods in managing constipation. We explore healthy fats, fermented foods, truths and myths about certain foods (bananas, anyone?), and the part played by high-fat diets, ultra-processed foods and eating habits.

Most of us are familiar with the importance of hydration, and Chapter 11 explains the role of fluids – water and others – in digestive health and constipation. It's all about what to drink and what to limit!

We take a look at behaviour in Chapters 12 and 13, starting in Chapter 12 with eating behaviour – where we suss out the timing of meals and how intuitiveness can help manage symptoms – and moving in Chapter 13 to the role of lifestyle. This includes the non-diet stuff that needs to be in your management strategies toolbox – helping you discover the connections between stress, movement and sleep – essentials that should be a part of your comprehensive management strategy.

In Chapter 14 we delve into the art of toileting, discovering the importance of optimal positioning and the gentle practice of bowel massage.

Chapter 15 cuts the wheat from the chaff to find out what are the 'yeas and nays' when it comes to the world of biotics – probiotics, prebiotics and more!

Chapter 16 sifts through the facts and myths surrounding laxatives, suggesting a ladder approach to their use, and even touches on the world of faecal microbial transplants and vibrating capsules!

The conclusion puts everything together, helping you see the bigger picture and encouraging you to compile your own transformation plan.

This book is for educational and informational purposes only.

This book does not replace personalised nutrition advice.

You should not use this information to diagnose or treat any health problems or illnesses without consulting your doctor.

It is recommended to seek advice from your doctor or consultant before making recommended changes.

Always seek the advice of your own doctor about your specific health situation.

•CHAPTER 1•
CONSTIPATION FRUSTRATIONS

Imagine this: in the hustle and bustle of the modern world, where our lives revolve around fast-paced routines and quick fixes, there exists a common gastrointestinal disorder that often goes unnoticed. For some people, even uttering the word can be challenging. This disorder, intertwined with a whole raft of potential dietary, medical and lifestyle triggers, and with its roots in both our culture and our environment, affects people in ways we might not fully grasp. This is the world of constipation, a topic often brushed aside yet deserving of attention and understanding.

Many of us have experienced constipation at some point. While some can shrug it off as a minor inconvenience, others may find it considerably more problematic. The reality is that constipation is a quiet but very determined troublemaker in one's digestive system. It is, in fact, very common, with most reports indicating that 15 per cent or at least one in seven people are affected.

If your bowel habits once followed a seamless, predictable pattern only to suddenly start acting up, you're definitely going to notice the shift. And when you do, a little concern is totally in order. Constipation is also not just a story of discomfort. Its impact can extend far beyond the realm of physical sensations. It possesses the power to cast a long shadow on how you can function day to day.

As you delve into the pages of this book, you'll explore all the common facets along with the many idiosyncrasies of this condition. Constipation, like a chameleon, can manifest in many different guises. To make this book relevant to you, it's essential that you become familiar with your own constipation tendencies or any patterns, to help you implement the relevant practical solutions. Keep in mind that an official constipation assessment and diagnosis is the responsibility of your doctor. At the same time, learning more about how your constipation likes to express itself can help you identify the best solutions.

This book serves as a practical toolkit, offering straightforward tips for tackling mild to moderate constipation, and setting the foundation to resolve severe constipation. While these strategies will be beneficial for many, the nuanced nature of this condition means that some individuals might find themselves needing specialised medical attention for the best results. It's crucial to remember that personalised care, guided by a healthcare professional, is therefore a clever move.

Nevertheless, this book seeks to offer more than just a series of tips. It's designed to foster a deeper understanding and solution-focused foundation, setting you on a path to achieving long-lasting improvements. It's time to bridge the gap between healthcare expertise and everyday experiences! Managing the diagnosis and treatment of chronic constipation resembles piecing together a mosaic, and it's so important to recognise that each person will have their individual approach to assembling the pieces.

Know the lingo – the poo-nunciation of the action of moving one's bowels

The word 'constipation' – which doesn't sound in any way pleasant – has its origins in the Latin word 'constipare', which means to press or crowd together. The word evolved in meaning to refer to waste that becomes compacted in the bowel or intestine, and which results in difficult bowel movements. In the medical world, the terms 'defecation' and 'evacuation' may be used to describe the action of passing a bowel motion. 'Faeces' may be used to describe expelling waste. More common words are 'poo' and 'stools'. We are also all pretty familiar with 'number two', 'shit' or 'shite', 'dump', 'log', 'turd' and 'crap'. Throughout the ages, constipation has usually hidden behind these polite and impolite terms. In the pages of this book, the straightforward term 'stools' will be mostly used for clarity and candour.

Stigma and poo taboo

'Going for a poo' is an essential, natural process that helps our body eliminate waste. It's a universal human experience, yet, strangely, we often find it difficult to discuss. We can find stigma surrounding gut conditions including constipation in many societies, although its extent can vary. Despite growing interest in gut health and the crucial role of gut microbes in digestion – with some even willingly providing stool samples for testing – our bowel habits and constipation continue to be taboo and sensitive subjects.

That's fine if it's your personal preference. It just isn't helpful if you suffer and find it hard to talk about it. In such cases, keeping it a secret will just prolong the suffering and may delay your receiving the crucial help you need. Others may downplay the seriousness of their condition to avoid discussing it. The overall unease and hesitancy in openly discussing bowel movements likely originates from the widespread feeling of embarrassment, personal privacy and cultural norms associated with such conversations.

3

Take, for instance, how even from a young age we see bathroom banter often labelled off limits. Picture a family gathering, where young Johnny proudly announces the details of his successful bathroom victory that morning. The responses? Likely a blend of awkward giggles and hasty subject changes. In certain societies, even alluding to toilet activities may be considered socially inappropriate. Or, at a work lunch, Emily opens up about her constipation woes when on her work trip, when Sean chimes in about his impeccable regularity, and Anne ignorantly adds, 'You should just eat better and exercise more; it's not that hard!' Emily internalises these well-intentioned but dismissive comments, further intensifying her feelings of vulnerability and making her embarrassed to broach the topic again.

From sitcoms to the silver screen, the entertainment industry loves turning toilet troubles into viewing and comedy gold. For example, the famous chaotic bathroom scene in *Bridesmaids* comes to mind. If you've ever had to endure *The Boss Baby* movie, you'll remember when boss baby talks about his constipation and receives the overly exaggerated and grossly unhelpful reaction, 'Did something clog your Schnitzel chute?'! How can we forget *Trainspotting*'s 'worst toilet in the world' scene, where Renton is no longer experiencing heroin-induced constipation, or the laxative prank in *Dumb and Dumber*. All well and funny, but the unintended consequence of using humour is that people might underestimate the seriousness of bowel conditions, making talking about our bathroom experiences more intimidating.

For others, anything related to the toilet can bring up cringeworthy memories or feelings from past embarrassing moments. For example, imagine being Ruth, who at school accidentally farted loudly in front of her classmates. The unstoppable laughing and teasing that followed led to feelings of embarrassment and shame for Ruth. A loud fart – another one of our body's natural processes, with the average person farting about 14 times per day – is ultimately destined for ridicule and cruelty, reinforcing the stigma associated with bowel debris. Could breaking this silence improve the well-being of those affected by this often-ignored topic?

Is celeb advocacy breaking down taboos?

Over recent years, a surge of celebrities have been candid about their personal health struggles, and their vast influence can shatter health stigmas and foster a sense of solidarity among those with similar afflictions. They have included Selena Gomez sharing her mental health battles; Angelina Jolie heightening awareness of the genetic risks of breast cancer and destigmatising both the disease and the surgeries associated with its diagnosis; and Robert Downey Jr. speaking about his journey through substance abuse, relapse and recovery. Through their narratives, celebrities not only foster deeper understanding of their issues, but also provide a beacon of hope for many grappling with similar issues. Their stories underscore the power of visibility in driving societal change and encouraging open dialogue on subjects previously considered to be taboo.

A number of well-known individuals have openly acknowledged their struggles with irritable bowel syndrome (IBS), contributing to public awareness and understanding. Among these, Kurt Cobain provided a dark insight into his personal battle with the condition and its cruel impact on his life and career. High-profile figures such as Tyra Banks and Kourtney Kardashian have also spoken publicly about their experiences of IBS, with both contributing to the broader conversation around this often-stigmatised health issue, and hopefully encouraging others to seek help and support.

Unexpected constipation tales that have been circulated throughout the ages include the claim that Napoleon's loss at the Battle of Waterloo was due to constipation, and that Elvis Presley's death on the toilet was a result of a heart attack brought on by stools stuck in his bowel. While these stories have been debunked, if constipation was once considered good enough reason to explain the defeat of a formidable military leader and the untimely death of the King of Rock and Roll, then it's a condition worth talking about, right?

In more recent years, constipation caught the public's attention when Amy Schumer opened up about it during a chat with Oprah, which, given Oprah's stature, is significant. Another celebrated actress, Kristen Wiig, of *Bridesmaids* fame, candidly confessed at a Hollywood awards ceremony, 'I haven't pooped in four days—four days! Between travelling and nerves, and this tight dress, I'm genuinely getting worried.' This was an excellent and brave admission, and a highly relatable anecdote for constipation sufferers! Should more celebrities choose to discuss their experiences with constipation, considering it's likely that a similar percentage of them are affected as in the general population, this could contribute, even in a small way, to making the average person feel more at ease about addressing the topic.

Breaking the poo taboo: opening up about constipation

It is an accepted notion that once you have a better understanding of any health condition you will be less likely to feel stigmatised or embarrassed about it. This book aims to dispel myths, help you completely grasp how your gut works and provide accurate information, in the hope of reducing the tendency to view constipation as something to be ignored, or worse, as a personal failing. Understanding how common constipation is can help you realise that you are not alone in your experiences. It may even help you catch and address symptoms at an earlier stage, thereby reducing the costs of constipation, not just in terms of finances but also on your overall well-being.

Historical treatments

Throughout history, constipation has been a persistent medical challenge, with remedies ranging from ancient herbal concoctions to contemporary dietary approaches. One of the earliest records of constipation-related beliefs can be found in an Egyptian medical text, the Ebers Papyrus, which dates to the sixteenth century BC. This document suggests a theory that diseases result from toxins produced by decaying waste in the intestines – the infamous 'internal putrefaction' theory. This concept, which stayed around for only three thousand years, proposed that diseases could be traced back to internal putrefaction, the idea that undigested food can rot inside the body and cause health issues.

Fast forward to the nineteenth century, and a time when Europe developed a strong cultural emphasis on the idea that 'cleanliness is next to godliness'. This significantly shaped societal attitudes and practices regarding hygiene and sanitation. However, this belief went beyond just physical cleanliness. It pushed for purity in all aspects of life, including moral, spiritual and physical virtues in both one's internal self and one's external appearance. This was when we started to see the moral dimension of constipation – the prevalent belief that a 'clogged' body was seen as a sign of a morally tainted character.

As the nineteenth century progressed, advancements in medicine meant that our understanding of constipation became more nuanced, even if it was not always accurate. First the theory of 'intestinal autointoxication', which literally means self-poisoning, seen as an extension of the 'internal putrefaction' theory, proposed that toxins generated in the bowel could be absorbed into the bloodstream, contributing to a wide range of ailments. It actually gained popularity as it evolved into a widely used diagnosis for a multitude of disorders – those that baffled doctors at the time, including headaches, indigestion, impotence, nervousness and insomnia, as well as suicide, skin ailments, gum disease, tuberculosis, cancer and – believe it or not – spinsterhood!

Theories continued to evolve over time. For example, an influential Dr Lane suggested that when we evolved from walking on four legs to walking on two, our intestines became prone to gravitational challenges, causing constipation. He and others began to think modernisation might be having a negative impact on the colon's anatomy in urbanised populations, and attention turned towards less constipation with high-fibre diets. He famously commented that 'the whiter your bread, the sooner you're dead!'

The nineteenth century, a golden time for medical quackery, saw an explosion of so-called cures for constipation. The public's fears and anxieties about constipation fuelled a booming market for laxatives and other digestive remedies, with advertisements that were nothing short of marketing genius. One proclaimed, 'If you don't kill it, it will kill you!'; another, 'A little constipation will kill the strongest man – any man, any woman, any child'; and yet another showed a bottle of prune juice like a powerful horse pulling people in a cart, symbolising its ability to 'move the whole family'. Others cleverly disguised remedies in chocolate to appeal to youngsters. These ads reinforced the public belief that constipation was the root of nearly all disease, and emphasised the idea or belief that immediate purgation – regularly clearing out the body's digestive system – was the only remedy. Some took it even further, not just promising swift relief from constipation but also touting beauty enhancements, weight loss solutions and a variety of other glorious benefits.

Fascinatingly, the period also witnessed the introduction of unique devices like enema and colonic irrigation equipment. There was a multitude of patented medicines, and some bizarre inventions such as phallic-shaped intestinal brushes (yes, you would be alarmed!), supportive belts and deep abdominal massagers – which may have required the user to stand in a specific position or even inside the machine – became widely popular. The concept of surgery, especially colectomy (a surgical procedure in which all or part of the large intestine is removed) emerged as another sought-after treatment for autointoxication, for those in upper class circles, that is.

However, as scientific understanding progressed, experimental studies began to challenge the autointoxication theory. This eventually led to reduced acceptance among professionals in the 1920s. Instead, dietary recommendations began to take centre stage. Although misleading, yeast emerged as a widely endorsed dietary remedy, seen as a way to introduce friendly microscopic life into the colon. A more enduring recommendation came from Metchnikoff, often referred to as the father of probiotics, who discovered non-lactic microbes and led the way for the recognition of sour milk and yogurt as healthful foods for all manner of diseases.

High-fibre foods began trending as a response to the widespread belief that ill health stemmed from a lack of bulk in one's diet. As the consumption of refined foods – which had surged as a result of the phenomenal growth of the food processing industry in the late nineteenth and early twentieth centuries – was increasingly demonised, there was a significant introduction of bran-based breakfast cereals and breads, marketed to 'banish constipation'. A variety of bran-infused recipes, including bran biscuits, bran muffins and bran patties, became extremely popular. This widespread enthusiasm for bran and high-fibre foods was so intense that some referred to it as a national mania.

Medical professionals from this time, including Dr John Harvey Kellogg (yes, from Kellogg's cereals fame), began offering valuable advice on how to prevent constipation. Their recommendations included a diet rich in whole grains, fruits and vegetables, along with increased physical activity and heeding the body's call for a morning bowel movement. Interestingly, these recommendations were often considered quite challenging for the average person, asking for a level of self-discipline and effort that many weren't ready to embrace. When we look at the results of extensive population studies and observe Westernised diets today, it's remarkable how little things seem to have changed!

In today's world, our fascination with gut health not only persists, but is a mega trend, thanks to the spotlight on the study of the microbes (for example, bacteria) residing in our gut. The modern emphasis on fibre-rich diets, the continued popularity of cleansing and detox programmes, and the demand for laxatives all bear witness to the enduring legacy of our ancestors' preoccupations. As this book begins to delve into 'why you can't go', we continue this long-standing quest to understand and manage this digestive malady effectively.

Stuck in the stats

We now know that constipation is a common condition that transcends geographical boundaries, with an estimated one in seven people suffering at any one time. This suggests that approximately 800,000 individuals in Ireland could be experiencing constipation right now, making it an undeniably widespread issue. On top of these statistics, the prevalence of constipation becomes notably higher as people age, with 33 per cent of those aged 60 or older reporting occasional constipation. Among nursing home residents in Ireland, the percentage soars to 50 per cent. Constipation also appears to exhibit a somewhat higher prevalence among women.

But these are the official figures. The actual number of people with constipation may be underestimated, as at least 65 per cent of individuals experiencing constipation choose over-the-counter (OTC) laxatives instead of seeking immediate medical help. In other reports, 39 per cent dismiss constipation as a minor health concern. Unfortunately, a significant number express dissatisfaction with the treatments they've received, whether that was because they did not produce the desired results or because they caused unpleasant side effects. After all, nobody wants to go from dealing with stubborn constipation to experiencing an episode of uncontrollable diarrhoea! The stark reality is that for many, constipation is more than just a minor inconvenience; it can become a chronic condition, with up to 45 per cent of individuals enduring it for five years or longer. On top of that, unfortunately half of those who have encountered constipation are likely to experience it again.

Yes, we spend a crapload of money on constipation

Constipation's reputation extends beyond the human experience; it is also known in health economic circles. In the first year after being diagnosed with chronic constipation, people tend to spend an average of €310 on medical expenses. A significant portion of this expenditure – almost half – goes towards purchasing laxatives. Another quarter is allocated for hospital care, and the remaining quarter covers health issues related to constipation. In the UK, the cost of constipation has been shown to set the health service back a staggering £162 million, with over 50 per cent of this spent on laxatives (which excludes OTC laxatives), so the reality is that the total laxative spend is probably much higher. Constipation thus stands as a formidable player in medical costs, estimated to incur millions annually in Ireland too. So it's not only as a personal inconvenience, but as a societal issue, that it demands better understanding and management.

CHAPTER 2

THE DIGESTIVE SYSTEM

The Digestive Tract

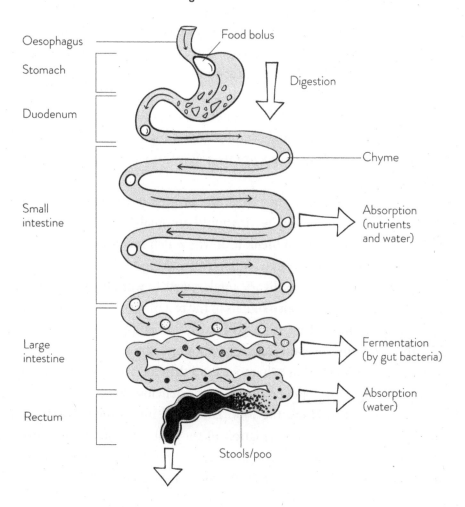

Oesophagus

Food bolus

Stomach

Digestion

Duodenum

Chyme

Small intestine

Absorption (nutrients and water)

Large intestine

Fermentation (by gut bacteria)

Absorption (water)

Rectum

Stools/poo

Understanding constipation becomes much easier when you have a grasp of how your extraordinary digestive system works. So, take some time out to understand the sophisticated steps that your amazing gut goes through as it transforms food into waste.

The journey to the large bowel

As we embark on our journey to the lower echelons of the gut, let's start by exploring how our digestive system responds to food even before we take our first bite. Our gut comes alive with anticipation at the mere hint of food, thanks to sensory cues such as the sight, smell and thought of food. This is known as the 'cephalic phase of digestion', when your brain signals to the gut to start to prepare for digestion. It results in the release of gastric juices in the stomach and enzymes in the pancreas. Your mouth produces saliva, often noticeable when you find yourself 'salivating' even before taking the first bite of food. This phase is your digestive system's way of warming up before you actually eat.

When you tuck into your food, the process of digestion logically begins in the mouth. Your teeth should automatically start working hard, chewing the food to break it down, which increases the surface area of the food. It also mixes it with saliva, making it easier for enzymes to act on it: in particular, salivary amylase gets to work breaking down carbohydrates. Chewing also signals to the rest of your digestive system that it's showtime, setting off a chain reaction and prompting things like the activation of pancreatic enzymes and the start of peristalsis, the wavelike motions that help move food through your digestive tract. It's fascinating what happens after just one delicious bite!

Finally, as you chew, the food is formed into a moist, ball-like mass called a bolus. The formation of the bolus is essential because it makes the food easier to swallow and facilitates its smooth passage from the mouth to the stomach. If food isn't chewed well, you could face some digestive challenges later, or at least your body will find it more difficult to extract and absorb nutrients.

Next in the journey, your meal embarks on a swift descent down the oesophagus, a muscular tube that connects your throat to your stomach. Once the food lands in your stomach, the volume of the food initiates a mechanical effect known as the 'gastric phase'. This makes your stomach adjust to its contents, and it also begins to secrete its powerful arsenal of stomach acids (including hydrochloric acid) and digestive enzymes, transforming your meal into a semi-liquid form known as chyme. There is then a controlled release of this chyme into the upper section of the small intestine, known as the duodenum.

Despite its misleading name, the small intestine measures around 6m in adults, making it much longer than the large intestine, which is thicker but only about 1.5m in length. The small intestine plays a major role in digesting food and absorbing nutrients. When nutrients are detected, the chemical breakdown begins with enzymes breaking down carbohydrates, proteins and fats into smaller, more manageable digestive molecules, and countless tiny, finger-like projections called villi and even smaller microvilli absorbing all the valuable nutrients released by the enzymes. The absorbed nutrients are then transported through the bloodstream to different parts of your body, providing energy, building materials (such as amino acids for muscle, for example) and everything else needed for the daily functioning of human beings.

Lastly, on average, approximately nine litres of fluid enters the duodenum – the first part of the small intestine – each day. This fluid comes from what you drink and the food you eat, but mostly from digestive juices produced by your body. As this fluid travels through the small intestine, it helps to mix and move the undigested food. By the time this mixture leaves the small intestine and heads into the large intestine, only about 1.5 to 2 litres of fluid remains. This remaining fluid, along with the undigested leftovers, continues down into the large intestine or colon. It usually takes around 5 hours for all of this to move through the small intestine, but it can vary from 2 to 7.5 hours.

The adventures of the large bowel (colon)

Next stop is the colon. The colon's primary role is to soak up water and shove the waste along, creating a perfect poo until it's time for it to leave the building. As more water is gradually absorbed back into the bloodstream, the waste material becomes more consolidated into stool. The cells lining the colon produce mucus, which helps lubricate the passage of poo. Along with water, the colon also absorbs essential salts, like sodium and potassium, and vitamins produced by the gut microbes.

The colon doesn't produce any enzymes, but its claim to fame is that it is teeming with trillions of magical microbes. These play a crucial role in breaking down dietary fibre and other components that enter the colon, essentially digesting what remains after initial digestion – our human leftovers. This process is believed to have a positive effect on digestion, which we'll explore in much more detail later in the book.

The large intestine is undoubtedly the epicentre of your digestive system when it comes to your stool getting through departures on time. If something is not working quite right, you will probably suffer the constipated effects. What's concerning is that the longer waste stays in the colon, the more water it absorbs, resulting in harder stools. How quickly or slowly food moves through the colon can change the types of bacteria there, which might change how the colon works. Other factors that might be at play are problems with certain cells or hormones within the large intestine. Or the muscles in the colon might not be working right. Sometimes, it's because people hold in their poo on purpose. Or for some it's not consuming enough of – or the right kind of – food or fluids. What could possibly go wrong?

Doing a poo

'Doing a poo' involves a sequence of clever interplays of automatic (things your body does without you thinking about it) and controlled (things you can consciously influence) functions in the end part of your colon. It's a team effort, where both your body's natural instincts and your conscious decisions work together. The rectum, which is the final section of the large intestine, connects the colon to the anus, the external opening at the end of the digestive tract. As the rectum fills with stool, it stretches, signalling to the body the need for a bowel movement. When the urge to empty is acted upon, the rectal walls should contract to expel the stool, and it passes into the anus. The rectum plays a critical role in the process of elimination, working in conjunction with the sphincter muscles at the anus to control and regulate the release of stools.

Unlike some animals that do their business wherever they happen to be, humans thankfully have conscious control over when and where they go! The process of doing a poo is firstly orchestrated by a network of neurons in the brainstem, often referred to as the defecation centre. Additionally, there is a relay and reflex centre in the lower spinal cord. Moreover, your body is impressively equipped with sensors that can differentiate between gas and stool. Think of it as a natural poo detector. So heading to the bathroom isn't just about convenience; it's the perfect example of your body's muscles and sensors working in harmony to ensure everything proceeds seamlessly.

When the stool reaches the anus, it signals that it's time to go. The anus is like the exit door. And just like a door can open and close, your anus can do the same to let the waste out when it's time to go. In the moments when you sense it's time, you'll typically sit down, take a deep breath, and gently relax the muscles in your diaphragm, abdomen and rectum. This coordinated effort is designed to aid the process, ideally leading to a smooth and comfortable bowel movement.

The act of doing a poo probably appears mundane to the casual observer, but it's undeniably quite a choreographed event. So the next time someone heads to the loo, maybe we can appreciate the extremely skilful processes happening behind closed doors!

The fascinating way the colon propels waste

The process of digestion in the colon hinges on two types of muscle contractions. Most of them (about 95 per cent) are peristalsis contractions, mixing the contents to help your body absorb water and salts. The remaining contractions push things forward. Some are slow and strong, while others are quick and light, with the faster ones playing a role in moving things along.

Additionally, there are high-amplitude propagated contractions, similar to wave-like motions. These are literally mass movements that complement peristaltic contractions by exerting strong, forceful waves of movement. They play a vital role in propelling substantial quantities of waste over longer distances in the colon, toward the rectum.

Now let's take a moment to appreciate an intriguing process called the gastrocolic reflex, which is one of your body's natural responses to eating. When you eat, your stomach stretches to make room for the food, and this stretching activates nerves that then send signals to the muscles in your large intestine, messaging to them to start contracting. This is your body's way of helping the digestion process along and getting the colon moving. It's like a gentle internal reminder that it's time to make space for the newly eaten food. The gastrocolic reflex plays a pivotal role in the functioning of the colon – in effect, by triggering these mass movements.

The colon's daily activity pattern generally shows an increase during the day, especially after meals, marked by these mass movements, when activated by the gastrocolic reflex. Occurring on average six times per day, mass movements are fundamental to regular bowel habits, as they provide the necessary force for the bulk movement of waste.

Furthermore, the colon's contractions are subject to signals from your nerves from the brain and spine. Hormones also play a role. For example, serotonin, acting as a neurotransmitter, acts like a director for your gut muscles, guiding the rhythm of their contractions. Then there's melatonin, beyond its role in sleep regulation, also working part-time to help synchronise the digestive system's daily rhythms.

The end is nigh

Apart from holding poo, the rectum has another important job. It has what's known as the 'rectal motor complex'. It's like a smart system that primarily moves in reverse to carefully control the flow of stool. Think of it as a built-in poo brake, which is especially handy at night. It makes sure that your rectum stays mostly empty until it's the right time for a bowel movement. How thoughtful of it!

As you can see, bowel movements are really the result of a fascinating interplay between muscle movements, nerve signals and hormonal cues, all responding in their own way to the foods we eat. This intricate system works like clockwork, and its efficiency – or any hiccups in it – can really impact the consistency of your stool and your bathroom habits, especially when it comes to constipation.

Total transit time

In people who don't have health issues, it takes anywhere from 24 to 72 hours from eating food to its passing out as stool. When scientists used a special kind of marker to see how long it took for food to travel through the colon, they noticed something surprising. Even in healthy people, this time could vary a lot over several months. A recent study found that the amount of water in a person's stool, which gives us a hint about gut travel time, can also change daily. This was true for both healthy folks and those with gut issues like IBS. So how quickly food moves through our gut can be as unpredictable as the weather, and a reminder that occasional changes in our bowel habits can be entirely normal. However, we should pay attention to more severe changes and not ignore them, just as we wouldn't ignore weather warnings!

Let's talk about poo, baby

We can produce a staggering amount of waste over the course of our lifetime – roughly equivalent to the weight of three small cars! Interested in discovering its contents? Time to investigate.

1. **Water:** About 74 per cent of what we excrete is water. The exact amount can vary depending on hydration and diet. Vegetarians tend to have more water, while those on a high-protein diet have typically less.

2. **Bacterial biomass:** What we excrete also includes a mix of microbes, both living and dead. It's estimated that 50 per cent are alive or, if you prefer, dead.

3. **Foodstuffs:** These include any undigested dietary fibre and other food remnants, including small amounts of fats and protein that the body didn't digest.

4. **Cells and waste products:** Cells that are shed from the lining of the intestines and other waste products from the body are also present.

5. **Bile pigments (bilirubin):** You will also find compounds produced by the breakdown of haemoglobin, which is the red pigment in blood cells. Bilirubin, which gives your stool its brown colour, is a by-product of the breakdown of haemoglobin in red blood cells.

6. **Inorganic substances:** These include trace elements such as calcium phosphate and iron phosphate.

Bowel movements differ greatly in terms of their appearance and characteristics, influenced by various factors that add a touch of uniqueness to each one, such as dietary choices, bodily functions and personal routines, especially for those dealing with constipation. Here are some more interesting facts about them.

What's the frequency norm?

Contrary to what you may think, everyone has a different pooing schedule, and our bodies are wonderfully diverse, meaning that everyone's digestive rhythm is unique to them. There's a common misunderstanding out there, and it's about thinking that you absolutely *must* have a daily visit to the bathroom. This belief sometimes causes people to consider less frequent bathroom trips as constipation. For instance, some elderly individuals with a normal bowel frequency – that is, more than three times a week – have been shown to perceive themselves as constipated if not moving their bowels once a day, and they consequently turn to laxatives. But the truth is that what's normal can vary from person to person.

For most healthy adults, the '3 and 3' rule is often mentioned, which means that anywhere from three bowel movements per day to three bowel movements per week is perfectly fine. So, having somewhere between 3 and 21 bowel movements a week falls within the wide range of what's considered normal.

The Bristol Stool Chart

The Bristol Stool Chart, developed by UK doctors in 1997, provides a useful visual guide to different stool shapes. It allows you to simply point and say, 'Yes, that's what my stool looks like!', without the need to provide a physical sample. Maybe we could start a petition to expand the poo emoji's repertoire and make it even more representative of our diverse digestive experiences. After all, emojis are all about expressing ourselves.

The visual aid presents seven distinct types of poo, each depicted with explanatory pictures and meaningful descriptions:

Bristol stool form scale

Type 1 Severe constipation		Separate hard lumps, hard to pass
Type 2 Mild constipation		Sausage-shape, but lumpy
Type 3 Normal		Like a sausage, but with cracks on its surface
Type 4 Normal		Like a sausage or snake, smooth and soft
Type 5 Lacking fibre		Soft blobs with clear-cut edges
Type 6 Mild diarrhoea		Fluffy pieces, mushy stool
Type 7 Severe diarrhoea		No solid pieces, entirely liquid

Type 1 or type 2 stools are the constipated types, whereas types 3 and 4 are normal and types 5 to 7 are on the looser end of the scale. The type of stool can also serve as an index of transit time in the digestive system. For example, types 1 and 2 are different severities of hard and lumpy stools, which can suggest a slower transit time.

Stool colour

Stool comes in a rich array of colours. From shades of brown to the occasional green or even red, the colour can be influenced by your diet, medication and sometimes underlying health conditions. Understanding this colourful spectrum can be a key to decoding your body's signals.

For the record, all shades of brown and even green are considered normal. As mentioned, the colour of stool is influenced by bile pigments and the breakdown of haemoglobin, which play a role in giving poo its brown colour. Changes in stool colour, such as pale stools or dark stools, can indicate underlying medical conditions. Bleeding in the colon can turn your poo red, while upper gastrointestinal bleeding may cause them to be black, as a result of bacterial breakdown of blood. Consuming foods like beets or food dyes can also temporarily make poo red.

Should your poo sink or swim?

Healthy stools typically sink in the toilet. You see, it's all about what's inside – the water, fibre, bacteria and waste products. Stools with more water are heavier or denser, and so tend to sink to the bottom. On the other hand, stools with less water might decide to float on the surface. What if you discover floating stools? Well, it isn't a cause for immediate panic. Occasionally, it can happen to the best of us because of factors like gas trapped in the stool or certain dietary choices, particularly those rich in fibre and occasionally those high in fat or alcohol, which can make your stools more buoyant. So, if you ever find your stool defying gravity, it's not necessarily a sign of trouble. Things should eventually settle back at the bottom of the bowl, just like they usually do.

So I hope you agree that what enters your toilet can tell a lot about your health. Imagine a future where 'smart toilets' could do the analysing for us. These advanced toilets, currently in the research and development phase, are being designed with sensors and artificial intelligence algorithms to examine the physical and chemical makeup of your stool, such as its shape, consistency and colour, and any signs of blood or unusual substances. They might even be able to analyse the microbes in your stool or microbiome, so they hold exciting potential for better understanding and managing conditions like constipation.

If you notice ongoing changes in how your stool appears, like dealing with constipation, diarrhoea or a mix of both (types 1, 2, 5, 6, or 7), unusual colours, blood in the stool, or stools that seem to have a mind of their own and float, it's a good idea to chat with a healthcare professional. These shifts might be signalling something going on in your gut or related to your diet, and getting expert advice can help put your mind at ease and get things back on track.

• CHAPTER 3 •

WHAT IN THE CONSTIPATION IS GOING ON?

In medical speak, constipation is referred to as a heterogeneous disorder, which means that it isn't just one straightforward problem with a single cause or symptom. Instead, it's a complex issue with a range of causes and manifestations. The symptoms and experiences people have vary enormously. Some might have infrequent bowel movements, while others might have hard stools or difficulty passing them. Others might be constantly bloated and feel nauseous. It really depends! And as you continue reading, you will realise that it's not just a basic bowel issue. It intertwines with our daily habits, the mechanics of our digestive system and our emotional state.

Consider constipation as a web of intrigue with many interconnected strands. To find a solution from a web, you need to start by identifying the central point or issue and then trace outwards, following each strand to understand its connection and significance to the main problem. This is the best way to discover how to get your personal plumbing unstuck. Every strand is covered in this book.

Constipation diagnosis

Many individuals have misconceptions about what is considered a regular bowel pattern. Surprisingly, almost a third of individuals who denied being constipated actually meet the criteria for chronic constipation! It's a common occurrence at the Gut Health Clinic to come across people who are unaware of their constipation. When asked about their problems, most will mention symptoms such as bloating, flatulence, pain, fatigue and headaches – indeed, symptoms of constipation – but not the condition itself! This underscores the need for all of us to sharpen our awareness of the telltale signs and symptoms of constipation.

In addition, those who *do* recognise that they have constipation often describe it based on the discomfort they feel during bowel movements, the need to strain, or the passage of hard stools, while doctors tend to define it more specifically as infrequent bowel movements. This difference in perspective can cause confusion and result in some constipation cases being overlooked or not recognised by individuals themselves.

It might come as a surprise that sometimes the real reason behind constipation is a bit of a mystery. But fear not! Doctors have an effective way to figure things out. A thorough examination of your medical history, coupled with a constipation assessment known as the Rome criteria checklist, usually suffices to help define your issues. These can help understand gut issues when regular medical tests often can't find a clear physical or organic cause for them – which in most cases is constipation and IBS. These Rome criteria have been developed by global experts, in Rome, and are updated every 6 to 10 years. Rome IV is the current version.

Diagnosing constipation

According to the Rome IV criteria, an individual is classified as experiencing constipation if they exhibit two or more of these symptoms at least 25 per cent of the time, with the symptoms lasting for a minimum of three months and having started at least six months before the diagnosis:

• struggling or straining during bowel movements

• passing hard or lumpy stools (see types 1 and 2 above on the Bristol Stool Chart)

• sensation of incomplete evacuation – a feeling like not everything has been eliminated or passed

• feeling an obstruction or blockage preventing stool passage

• requiring the use of hands or assistance to have a bowel movement

• having fewer than three spontaneous, unassisted bowel movements in a week

• not experiencing diarrhoea, unless prompted by interventions like medication

• lacking the typical symptoms of IBS.*

* Constipation and IBS are two distinct conditions. See IBS diagnosis criteria on page 34.

Always remember, while this book offers guidance, it's essential to chat with your doctor about any constipation concerns. Don't be tempted to self-diagnose!

The visit to the doctor's office

To uncover the mystery behind your persistent constipation, doctors will need to take a look at your medical history, ask you a range of personal questions and of course conduct a detailed physical exam. To help define constipation, they will want to find out more.

For example, they will ask if you've had surgeries or any known conditions – like thyroid problems, diabetes or depression – that might affect going to the bathroom. They will want to know what medications you take.

Once that background check is out of the way, put on your storytelling hat and get ready to share your once-upon-a-time constipation story.

Questions your doctor may ask:

- *Poo:* What is your 'normal'? How often do you go, what does it look like (look at the wonderful pictures on the Bristol Stool Chart to pick your number(s)) and/or do you have to push hard or strain to get it out?

- *Sensations:* How do you feel after doing a poo – do you feel empty and relieved, or do you feel your bowel has not emptied completely?

- *Blood:* Is there any blood in your poo – how much, and for how long has this been happening?

- *Hands:* Do you use little tricks like pressing certain areas down there to help the poo come out?

- *Laxatives and supplements:* Do you use laxatives or enemas, including at-home versions – how much and for how long?

- *Other:* What do you eat, what are your daily routines, are there any substances you might be using, or have you experienced any major life events (like childbirth, or bereavement or other trauma), and what are your stress levels like day to day?

Digging into these possible causes can hint at why you might be having constipation. Opening up about your bowel habits will help bring clarity to the situation. On the other hand, holding back may hinder the doctor's ability to grasp the complete picture. So why not do yourself a favour and share openly and freely?

The physical exam

Think of a physical exam as a detective taking a close look at the scene of the crime – scoping out the back-door area. Your doctor inserts a gloved, lubricated finger, first peeking outside and then venturing inside to ensure everything's in order. In what's called a digital rectal exam, they're checking for any unwanted guests. By examining the exit (anus and rectum), doctors can check to see how things move when you try to poo, and feel for any lumps or issues like haemorrhoids, small tears or blockages. They can also get a feel for what's inside, feeling the muscle tone to see if there's any poo stuck up there. Furthermore, misbehaving pelvic floor muscles can be detected. They may also feel your belly to see if there are any unusual lumps.

It's not as scary as it seems!

If the idea of a physical exam feels a bit daunting, you're not alone. It's perfectly normal for people to get nervous about the idea of someone putting a finger up their bum – from cultural taboos, personal embarrassment, the fear of the unknown and medical stigma. It's all very understandable. However, try to remember a few things:

- *It's routine for doctors:* For your doctor, conducting a physical exam is as routine as Darina Allen making her soda bread. They've done it so often and they will always aim to make it as comfortable as possible for you.

- *Your comfort is a priority:* Let your doctor know if you're anxious. They can explain every step beforehand so there are no surprises and you know what to expect.

- *It's a crucial step to better health:* Avoiding or postponing a physical exam because of anxiety can delay finding out the root of the issue. The sooner you get checked, the quicker you can get on the path to feeling better.

- *You're in control:* If at any point you feel uncomfortable or want to stop the exam, it's okay to say so. Your doctor is there to help and work with you.

While the idea of a physical exam might seem intimidating, it's a short process that can provide a wealth of information. It's always better to face it head-on than to be left wondering what's causing your discomfort. Your bowel is worth it.

Recognising red flags in chronic constipation

Remember, you're not alone in this, and recognising anything outside the norm is just a sensible way of taking proactive steps for your well-being. To make a diagnosis, doctors will make sure there's none of these warning signs, which sometimes signal something more serious:

- *Unintentional weight loss, more than 10 per cent over 3 months:* For example, if you weigh 10 stone and you find yourself shedding a whole stone without even trying in just 3 months, it's considered a signal that you should talk to your doctor.

- *Blood in your stool:* This means that your poo will appear either a bright red or a dark and tarry colour. This *can be* related to more serious gut problems, including haemorrhoids or inflammation, and is therefore worth checking out.

- *Nocturnal bowel movements:* This refers to the urge to have bowel movements during the night. Typically, the body's body clock or circadian rhythms align bowel movements with daytime hours, so it's unusual to be awakened from slumber to move one's bowels.

- *Sudden, severe constipation in people over 50:* If you experience a sudden and severe onset or worsening of constipation, it's a reason to chat with your GP.

- *Family history of colorectal cancer, IBD or coeliac disease:* While not a direct cause of constipation, this genetic trait can make some people or their family members more likely to have gut issues, so it's worth getting it checked out.

- *Abnormal blood work such as anaemia:* Anaemia or iron deficiency is a condition where the body lacks enough iron to produce sufficient red blood cells. Constipation along with anaemia can indicate underlying issues such as internal bleeding in the digestive tract.

If you notice any of these warning signs, again, don't put it off – consult your doctor. They can investigate further and determine the underlying cause. If this makes you feel anxious or worried, remember that it's always better to be proactive than sorry. Your health is your wealth, and catching potential problems in the early stages can make a big difference. While these signs may point to a serious issue, they don't always mean there *is* a major problem. Think of them as a heads-up that prompts you to get the right help. Is it constipation, or is it something else? The more details you can provide, the better your doctor can help.

Additional diagnostic tests

If there are red flags from your medical assessment, more tests might be needed. People who still have constipation even after trying regular treatments might also need extra tests that may include:

- *Blood tests:* Blood tests don't hold much value in pinpointing constipation directly. This is because most types of constipation are devoid of physical or biochemical changes. Blood tests may be recommended to check things like your overall blood health – for example, thyroid function, blood sugar level, inflammation or infection.

- *Abdominal ultrasound:* This test uses sound waves to create pictures of the inside of your belly. It can show inflammation, unusual structures in the digestive system or growths.

- *X-rays:* Simple X-ray images of your abdomen can show if there's a blockage in your intestines.

- *Barium enema:* This test helps doctors see issues like an unusually large colon or rectum. Sometimes, a barium enema is used with X-rays to get a clearer view of the colon.

- *Colonoscopy:* This test lets doctors look directly inside your colon. It's often done if you have warning signs or other symptoms. It's a way to check for unusual changes in the colon.

In the realm of medical diagnostics, you may also stumble upon a collection of peculiarly named specialised tests. Depending on the unique tale your symptoms tell, how you respond with treatments and the available testing centres, some of these may also be considered:

- *Balloon expulsion test:* Here, a tiny balloon is placed in the rectum and filled up with water, and then you're asked to try to push it out. This can show if there are challenges with the normal process of passing stool.

- *Colonic transit time measurement:* This is a fancy way to say 'how long it takes for food to move through your colon'. There are a few ways to measure this, including special markers that show up on X-rays or a tiny wireless capsule that reports on the time it takes. This helps tell if things are moving too slowly or if there's a problem with the pelvic floor muscles.

- *Anorectal manometry:* These tests check how well your anus and rectum work. They measure things like the pressure in your anal sphincter, how your rectum responds when you strain or cough and your sensitivity to sensations. It's pretty good at spotting issues like muscle problems at the end of your bowel and is becoming more advanced with 3D imaging technology.

- *Defecography:* This is a study of your body's mechanics during a bowel movement. In this unique X-ray procedure, a contrast material is gently inserted into your rectum. You'll be asked to simulate a dummy bowel movement while the radiographer captures X-ray images, all displayed on a screen (and who is not looking at you!). These images provide a real-time view of how your rectum and anus function, allowing them to observe your muscles and organs in action and identify any physical changes that might contribute to constipation.

Choosing the right test requires a tailored approach. Sometimes, when basic solutions like tweaking daily habits or trying OTC laxatives don't do the trick, or if there are signs that make the doctor more concerned, more specific tests might be needed.

Types of constipation

To unravel the complexities of constipation and enhance treatment approaches, experts have constructively categorised it into two main subtypes, primary and secondary constipation, with further classifications within these subtypes for added clarity. Most people find themselves in the 'primary constipation' club, which means their symptoms match up with the Rome IV criteria. On the flip side, if constipation tags along because of another medical issue or medication, it's called 'secondary constipation'.

Primary causes	Secondary causes
Normal transit constipation IBS-constipation Slow transit constipation Evacuation disorder Mixed primary types	Medications Medical conditions

Primary constipation

Normal transit constipation

Normal transit constipation is the most common type, accounting for roughly half of all reported constipation cases. It's also puzzling because it doesn't have an apparent underlying cause. In the medical world, this mysterious condition is referred to as 'idiopathic' constipation.

People with this type of constipation often complain of infrequent bowel movements, hard or lumpy stools, and a sense of incomplete evacuation. Despite these symptoms, tests and examinations often reveal no abnormalities in the gastrointestinal tract. Food and waste move through the large intestine at a normal speed.

Irritable bowel syndrome with constipation (IBS-C)

Irritable bowel syndrome (IBS) is a common digestive disorder characterised by various gut-related issues. Despite its prevalence, the exact causes and mechanisms of IBS are not fully understood either! IBS with constipation (IBS-C) is a type of irritable bowel syndrome where the main issue is ongoing abdominal (tummy) pain along with constipation. Interestingly, just like with normal transit constipation, the way things move through the colon again usually falls within the normal range for most people with this type of constipation, although IBS-C gets its own distinct set of Rome IV criteria.

Diagnosing IBS-C

Frequent abdominal or stomach pain which happened at least one day per week in the last three months, and which started at least six months ago.

The stomach pain is related to at least two of the following:

- having a bowel movement (can make it better or worse)
- changes in how often you have a bowel movement
- changes in how to the stools look
- having more 'hard or lumpy' bowel movements than 'loose or watery' ones.

Other symptoms:

- straining during bowel movements
- feeling like you haven't completely emptied your bowels
- feeling like there's a blockage in your bowel passage.

In the case of IBS, which is now recognised as a disorder involving the interaction between the gut and the brain, again standard medical tests typically do not reveal any underlying physical causes for these symptoms. And in case you need to hear this – it's not all in your head. The symptoms are 100 per cent real and valid.

However, while healthcare professionals use the Rome criteria to try to tell constipation and IBS-C apart, it can be quite tricky in practice, as these conditions often share many of the same symptoms, and the division between them is often blurred. The main difference is that pain is not a diagnostic symptom for constipation, whereas pain *is* a diagnostic symptom for IBS-C.

Interestingly, a study revealed that nearly 90 per cent of IBS-C patients also display symptoms of constipation. Conversely, around 44 per cent of constipation patients fulfil the criteria for IBS-C! Understanding that constipation and IBS-C share a lot of similar symptoms helps, because it further shows how these conditions are complex. In contrast to individuals dealing with mild constipation, those experiencing severe pain often report more pronounced physical discomfort, a reduced sense of well-being and a greater impact of bowel issues on their daily life.

Slow transit constipation

Slow transit constipation is a less prevalent manifestation of constipation, but can be highly challenging. Historically, it has been referred to as colonic inertia, where your colon isn't doing a good job of pushing stool out of your body when you need to go to the bathroom. It affects about 15 per cent of those who are regularly constipated. Those with slow transit constipation have more infrequent bowel movements, often less than once a week.

This can happen when the muscles in your colon aren't cooperating as they should, which can affect peristalsis, the coordinated muscle contractions that move stool through the intestines. The consequences of delayed colonic transit and motility issues can include inadequate squeezing and the inability to move things forward, leading to increased tightness, a relaxed end part of the bowel, or even backward movements within this region. Another thing to consider is that your pelvic floor muscles and your colon should work well together (more on this below); if they're not, this can slow down how things move in your gut.

Recent research suggests other factors that may be at play. These may include some interesting changes in what are known as the interstitial cells of Cajal. Think of these cells as the pacemakers of your intestines. There might also be some tweaks in the number or structure of nerve cells in the gut, as well as some unusual patterns in the intestinal muscle fibres. While the exact effect of these changes on constipation has not yet been figured out, it's clear they play a role in how things work.

The consequences of slow transit constipation are that when the stool stays in your large intestine or colon for a long time, your body will continue to absorb water from it, making it smaller and harder, which will usually lead to more abdominal discomfort. Increasing your fibre intake may not always provide the relief you hope for, because things can get more backed up. But don't worry; it doesn't necessarily mean you need to switch to a low-fibre diet. Trying to make your stool softer, like most people aim to do with constipation, can be beneficial. However, slow transit constipation is a condition that should be effectively evaluated and managed by your healthcare team to find the best approach and provide hope for improvement.

Defecation disorders

Defecation disorders refer to difficulties in having a bowel movement, which can lead to constipation. These include alien-sounding diagnoses like defecation dyssynergia and anorectal dysfunction. These are linked to problems involving the pelvic floor muscles, which are the muscles located around the end of your bowel, and they play a crucial role in controlling your bowel movements. These muscles are the puborectalis and the external and internal anal sphincter muscles.

Ultimately, defecation disorders result in inadequate bowel motions. People typically report excessive straining when trying to move their bowels, and they experience a sensation of bowel blockage and quite frequently the feeling of incomplete evacuation. Moreover, prolonged straining during defecation can lead to the weakening of pelvic floor muscles, elevating the risk of structural abnormalities and other complications. These issues can be seen in 25 to 30 per cent of people with constipation.

Symptoms often make their debut in childhood, and a substantial number of individuals who experience childhood constipation continue to struggle with these challenges into adolescence and beyond. It can also affect women who have recently given birth, and older people.

Why this happens is usually unclear. These uncoordinated responses could be triggered by factors such as pain, a previous surgery, or a history of trauma. Sometimes, the cause of defecation difficulties stems from neurological issues, such as those seen in spinal cord injuries, nerve diseases such as multiple sclerosis (MS), or conditions like Parkinson's disease, where the nerve function that controls bowel movements can be compromised. Other times, slow stool movement through the colon is not directly due to the colon's function, but rather something impeding the flow, such as a pelvic floor prolapse or rectocele (when the wall of the rectum bulges into the back wall of the vagina).

In many cases, specific problems with your nerves or body structure are not responsible. If this is the case, you may be given a diagnosis of a 'functional defecation disorder', which means the trouble comes from how your body works rather than from something physical that is wrong.

It's important to recognise when something's amiss with your bathroom habits. If you find that you can't fully empty, feel like something's obstructing your stool, experience prolonged bathroom visits, frequently need to strain, or need to resort to using your hand to assist, it could be a sign of a potential exit issue. Additionally, if you've followed dietary, lifestyle and laxative advice without seeing the desired results, it's a significant hint that your pelvic floor might be playing a role in your unsatisfactory bowel movements.

Trying to identify the specific mechanisms causing these disorders is essential for optimising treatment. For this, the expertise of a pelvic health physiotherapist is invaluable. These highly skilled physios are like magicians when it comes to pelvic health. They possess a deep understanding of the intricate workings of the pelvic floor muscles and the complex interactions within the pelvic region. With their knowledge and specialised techniques, they can work wonders in diagnosing and treating issues related to pelvic floor dysfunction. In addition, to figure out what the root cause is, doctors may need to use specialist tests like anorectal manometry and defecography (explained on page 32) to help further understand why this is happening.

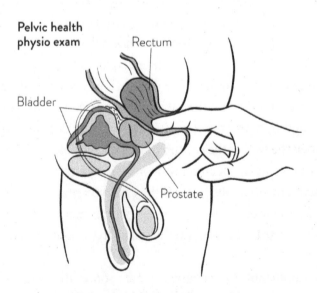

Pelvic health physio exam

Summary, primary constipation

In summary, primary constipation can arise from multiple mechanisms, including normal transit constipation, IBS-C, slow colonic transit, and defecation disorders. Figuring out what's causing the constipation is going to help in choosing the right treatment that targets the root of the problem. And just to throw a spanner in the works, it's important to keep in mind that everyone's experience with constipation and response to treatments can vary widely. While some individuals dealing with normal transit constipation might see improvement with simple diet and lifestyle adjustments, these approaches may only provide partial relief for those dealing with slow transit constipation. For individuals with defecation disorders, incorporating dietary changes can be beneficial, but it's often essential to seek specialised care from a pelvic health physiotherapist for more comprehensive management. Stay tuned for later in the book, where we'll delve deeper into these topics and provide valuable insights and guidance for managing constipation effectively.

Exploring secondary constipation and its causes

Secondary constipation is typically associated with an underlying medical condition or medications.

Medical conditions

Secondary constipation, sometimes called organic constipation, happens because of other diseases that affect the functioning of your colon, rectum or anus. These diseases can be quite varied and include:

- *Structural issues or blockages:* This can happen as a result of scar tissue (adhesions), cancer, narrow areas (strictures), or the pressure from other body parts or unusual growths in the abdomen.

- *Gastrointestinal conditions:* Conditions such as inflammatory bowel disease (IBD), small intestinal bacterial overgrowth (SIBO), diverticulosis or colorectal cancer can cause changes in bowel habits, including constipation.

- *Metabolic issues:* These include conditions such as an underactive thyroid (hypothyroidism), diabetes and too much calcium in the blood (hypercalcaemia).

- *Neurological disorders:* These include diseases that affect the nerves and brain, like Parkinson's disease or multiple sclerosis.

- *Other whole-body conditions:* Conditions such as scleroderma (a disease that hardens the skin and connective tissues) or amyloidosis (where abnormal levels of protein build up in organs) can lead to constipation.

- *Hormonal changes:* Fluctuations in hormone levels, particularly during pregnancy, can lead to constipation in some individuals.

- *Psychological conditions:* Mental health issues like depression or eating disorders can also lead to constipation.

In cases where constipation is linked to a specific health condition, addressing the root cause often alleviates the constipation as well. It's essential to consult with a healthcare professional who can accurately diagnose and treat the underlying issue.

Medications

Several medications can disrupt normal bowel movements, leading to constipation as an unwanted side effect. If it's determined that specific medications are contributing to constipation, healthcare professionals might look into modifying or stopping these drugs when it's safe and practical to do so. This approach helps manage constipation while ensuring overall medical treatment remains effective.

For example, painkillers, especially opiates and some medications used for nerve pain or epilepsy, are notorious for causing constipation.

If you need these medications and are struggling with constipation, you might need to switch to another pain reliever or add a laxative to counteract constipation.

Some medications, including blood pressure drugs, older anti-depressants like tricyclics, iron supplements, heartburn medications like antacids, as well as medications for Parkinson's disease, seizures and psychological conditions, can lead to constipation. This can happen because these medications affect muscle activity, nerve signals or gut motility. It's good to stay informed and have a conversation with your doctor if you think you are experiencing an increase in constipation due to medication.

Potential consequences of chronic constipation

While constipation may seem harmless at first glance, it can evolve into a persistent condition with the potential for serious complications, including:

- *Haemorrhoids:* Commonly known as piles, haemorrhoids are swollen blood vessels in the rectum or anus that can be painful and often lead to rectal bleeding. Repeatedly exerting force to expel stool can cause or worsen them, likely because of the added pressure inside the abdomen affecting the blood vessels.

- *Anal fissures:* Anal fissures are small tears in the lining of the anus, typically resulting from the passage of large or hard stools, straining, reduced blood flow to the area, and issues with the anal sphincter.

- *Rectal prolapse:* Pushing hard and often during bowel movements can lead to part of the rectum slipping out of its normal position and protruding from the anus. Symptoms of rectal prolapse include the feeling of a bulging from the anus, discomfort or pain in the rectal area, bleeding and difficulty with bowel movements.

- *Faecal incontinence:* This is when you can't control your bowel movements, and it might happen unexpectedly. It can vary from a little leak when you pass gas to more serious situations where you have no control at all. It's not something anyone likes to talk about, but it can affect your daily life and how you feel emotionally.

At times, the challenges associated with moving one's bowels can lead to more severe issues, such as:

- *Faecal impaction:* Faecal impaction is a condition where a large, solid mass of hard, dry stool gets stuck in the rectal waiting room. This condition often occurs in individuals who have been constipated for an extended period of time. Factors such as an accumulation of poo, slowed bowel movement, and changes in sensitivity in the anus and rectum can contribute to its development.

Symptoms you should not ignore

If you haven't had a bowel movement for three days and you're experiencing any of the following symptoms, it's important to get in touch with your healthcare provider:

- Nausea (feeling sick)
- Vomiting
- Sensation of fullness after consuming liquids
- A sensation of 'tightness' in your abdominal region
- Persistent bloating and swelling in the abdominal area.

These signs might suggest something needs attention, and it's a good idea to chat with your doctor about it sooner rather than later. Your comfort matters!

Constipation and overflow diarrhoea

Did you know that you can have diarrhoea and be constipated at the same time? Although this may seem contradictory, it can occur. One of the reasons is a response known as 'overflow diarrhoea'. With this, for example, you would normally have type 1 stools (small, hard pellets), but now and again, out of the blue, you experience type 6 or type 7 stools (pretty much liquid). In this scenario, a person's intestines have become partially blocked because of the hard stool backing up in the bowel, or sometimes because there's a structural issue. As a result, some newer stool can bypass the blockage and leak around it, causing diarrhoea-like symptoms.

Picture the digestive system as a dam, with the hard stool serving as the initial blockade. As time passes, softer and more liquid waste accumulates behind this obstacle, akin to water pooling behind the dam. Eventually, when the pressure reaches a breaking point, it swiftly forces the softer material to surge around and over the hard stool, often resulting in abrupt and unforeseen bowel movements, akin to a dam's wall finally yielding to the relentless force of the water it holds back. This can be quite surprising and understandably distressing for people.

The underlying cause of overflow diarrhoea is typically a prolonged history of constipation. It can be characterised by its unpredictability and inconsistency, as it may alternate with periods of severe constipation. If you are experiencing these symptoms, it's essential that you consult a healthcare provider for a thorough evaluation and appropriate management to address the underlying causes of both constipation and overflow diarrhoea.

Also, keep in mind that after a thorough 'clear-out' it might take a few days – maybe even up to three – for your regular stool to build up again. This could be why some folks notice a brief pause in their bowel movements after experiencing diarrhoea.

Further constipation punishment

A significant number of individuals who suffer from constipation also have to contend with an array of associated symptoms, which can reliably intensify the distress. Two of the primary symptoms often reported alongside constipation are flatulence and bloating, with or without distension.

Flatulence, or farting, is more than just a source of amusement. It's a result of the complex digestion of carbohydrates, which bacteria in our gut break down, producing gas. Most of these gases, including methane and carbon dioxide, don't have a smell. However, some, like hydrogen sulphide, are responsible for the infamous 'rotten egg' whiff of some farts. The food we eat, our unique gut bacteria and individual factors such as food intolerances all influence the amount and odour of our gas. Constipation can lead to increased flatulence, as the trapped stool in the colon can cause the production of more gas via the hungry microbes that are hanging out there.

We've all experienced a bloated feeling at some point in our lives. It's that uncomfortable sensation when your abdomen feels swollen and tight. Bloating often accompanies constipation and can be quite distressing. It occurs as a result of the build-up of gas or an increased sensitivity in the gut. The pressure from the trapped gas can leave you feeling full and uncomfortable and can even cause your belly to look swollen. Some people will also feel distended, which is the physical expansion of the abdomen. These symptoms are far from pleasant. But it's not just the physical discomfort that's bothersome. Bloating and distension can also affect your mood and self-confidence. You may find yourself avoiding social situations or feeling self-conscious about your appearance when bloating becomes noticeable. This emotional aspect of bloating adds an extra layer of frustration to the already challenging experience of constipation.

Common constipation-related symptoms

Although the symptoms people may experience if they have constipation can vary from person to person, they can include:

- flatulence

- bloating and distension

- fatigue

- nausea and sometimes vomiting

- loss of appetite, sometimes leading to malnutrition

- bad breath

- furred tongue

- reflux

- irritability

- poor sleep and, for some, insomnia

- increased stress and anxiety.

The potential list of symptoms is long and can contribute to a vague, indescribable sense of ill-health. In a very old experiment (one that would likely not receive ethical approval in today's research world), five healthy men were asked to not move their bowels for 90 hours (nearly 4 days). During this experiment, each man complained of symptoms such as a coated tongue, foul breath, mental sluggishness, headache, depression, restlessness, and irritability. Remarkably, all participants experienced immediate relief after receiving an enema (where a liquid is gently introduced into the rectum to soften and loosen stool and encourage bowel movements).

This experiment highlighted the relief that comes with moving your bowels and emphasised the importance of addressing constipation. Indeed, the relief can be utterly exhilarating when you successfully pass a normal bowel motion after experiencing constipation – you know that feeling, right?! This is a result of relief from the discomfort, pressure and other side effects that constipation can cause. It's a bit like a weight being lifted, both physically and emotionally. You feel physically lighter, more comfortable, and probably much happier! It's a reminder of the importance of healthy digestion and the role it plays in our overall well-being.

Impact of constipation on quality of life

The ripple effect of constipation on one's body can be significant and deeply disturbing, affecting one's quality of life (QOL). If not tackled, it can evolve and grow, further impacting your overall health and day-to-day existence. Along with the physical discomfort it exerts, it can take its toll on your personal life, work dynamics, social interactions and sex life. Mix in the emotional toll, and you're left with feelings of frustration and exhaustion.

Here are some common sentiments and comments that individuals might express when struggling with constipation:

'This relentless, gnawing pain in my stomach ... it's like a heavy weight pressing me down all day.'

'Everything I eat, everything I try ... nothing makes a difference.'

'It's too intimate, too embarrassing. How can I even mention it to my partner?'

'It's become my whole world, overshadowing everything else. I can't focus properly on anything.'

'The thought of being chained to laxatives for life? Unbearable.'

'This relentless pressure is wearing on my nerves. Why am I lashing out at everyone?'

'Should I stop eating, book a coffee enema, buy some detox tea, hang upside down? There has to be a way.'

'Could this be a sign of something worse ahead, like cancer?'

'Is it too much to ask? To just ... be like everyone else, and trot off to the loo and get the job done after my breakfast?'

'It's like I'm on an island, cut off. Does anyone else even know this pain?'

While these are just a few perspectives, it's essential to understand that everyone's experience with constipation is unique. From mild to moderate to severe, each person's journey is distinct and incomparable to another's. For many, it transcends physical unease, involving the emotional and psychological aspects of their lives.

Holding poo

At some point in our lives, we've all probably faced a situation where we've had to 'hold our poo'. A beautiful rose-smelling toilet, with soundproof privacy and soft, quilted toilet paper is not always in the vicinity. This challenge is real. However, once you locate a loo, even if it usually falls short of expectations, when the urge strikes, you should seize the opportunity.

Others may delay going to the toilet because of various inhibitions and concerns, such as embarrassment about smells or noise in public toilets. Occasionally, after an uncomfortable and emotionally distressing bathroom constipation session, some people might then delay their next visit to the loo to avoid repeating the ordeal.

According to medical experts, the occasional occurrence of holding is generally not a cause for concern. However, consistently delaying bowel movements can possibly increase constipation, as the longer stool remains in the colon, the drier and harder it becomes. It may also create a cycle where the natural reflexes and sensations associated with bowel movements get suppressed.

For example, if you make a habit of holding in your bowel movements too often, it can cause some unwelcome problems like tummy pain, bloating and excess gas. It may even lead to issues such as stretching your rectum, losing control over your bowel movements, painful haemorrhoids, anal tears, or even getting stool stuck, which would need medical help. So it's best not to delay those bathroom trips.

In the grand scheme of things, for the sake of your bowel it's a good idea not to make a habit of holding in your poo. That's why one of the golden rules in the world of digestive issues is to listen to your body's signal for a bathroom break – the 'call of nature' – and act on it when it comes knocking. You can dive deeper into this topic in Chapter 14, which deals with 'toileting tricks'.

Risk factors for constipation

Chronic constipation typically arises from a complex combination of various risk factors and lifestyle decisions. Understanding and addressing these elements, when possible, is key to both preventing and effectively managing constipation. Here are some of the critical factors that appear to be closely linked with the occurrence of constipation.

Age and gender

As we touched on earlier, age plays a significant role in the risk of chronic constipation, especially as we get older. This may be because, with our taste buds changing, we might not eat as much fibre-rich food or stay as hydrated as we used to. In addition, we may be taking more medications as we age that can unintentionally cause constipation. Things like dentures, tooth loss and difficulty chewing might lead older individuals to prefer softer, low-fibre foods, which could also contribute to the issue. Age-related changes in the body's structure, like rectal and pelvic floor changes, can also be factors.

Now, let's talk about the gender aspect. Constipation rates are higher in women than in men, although the exact reasons aren't entirely clear. Hormonal fluctuations during pregnancy and the changes that happen in the perimenopausal years can disrupt bowel regularity. Women's pelvic floor muscles and nerves can also be affected by childbirth, which could end up being the link to constipation. On top of that, women tend to be more proactive in dealing with constipation, often reaching for laxatives and seeking medical help. Lastly, women's higher participation in research studies can inevitably make it tricky to fully understand these gender differences.

Poor dietary choices

Let's talk about diets and their impact on constipation. The typical Western diet, with its high amount of fat and refined sugars, excessive salt, and limited fruits, veggies and fibre, isn't exactly a friend to your bowels. On the flip side, the Mediterranean diet, which is packed with plant-based foods and healthy fats, seems to have all the attributes to be a constipation-busting superstar. In addition, those who follow a vegetarian or vegan diet tend to have more regular bowel movements than do those who eat more meat and less fibre.

Now fibre is obviously going to be in the spotlight when it comes to managing constipation, but it's not the sole culprit or saviour. In fact, the role of dietary fibre in constipation isn't entirely clear-cut. Surprisingly, around 80 per cent of people in Ireland don't get enough fibre, yet the constipation rate isn't nearly as high. This suggests there's more to the story. Some folks with chronic constipation actually have similar fibre intakes to those without it, and increasing fibre can even make things worse for some. It's a bit of a puzzle!

But getting enough fibre is generally a good idea for managing constipation and keeping your gut happy. There is more on the best types of fibre foods, how much of them to eat, and how to incorporate them effectively in Chapters 6 and 7.

Dehydration

Inadequate water intake is frequently linked to constipation, and this is true. Dehydration will elevate the likelihood of you experiencing constipation. More on this in Chapter 11.

Physical inactivity

When it comes to how physical activity plays into constipation, some research suggests that moderate exercise might help reduce the chances of getting constipated, but there are also studies with different findings. While we often think that being too inactive, like being stuck in bed for a while, could lead to constipation, the proof for this isn't rock solid. So, in a nutshell, the connection between physical activity and constipation is a bit fuzzy. More on this in Chapter 13.

Social and economic influences

Life's challenges can bear a heavier burden on those in less fortunate situations, and even something as simple as constipation can tie into these larger struggles. Things like money issues, not having many healthy food choices around, living in stressful conditions, or relying on specific medications can all mess with your digestion. It's important to know that it's not always about making bad food choices. Sometimes, it's just not having easy access to good food. If we push for better healthcare access and try to understand everyone's unique stories, we can help cut down on these health problems and make life better for everyone.

Anorexia, disordered eating and undereating

For individuals facing challenges like restricted eating or who are coping with eating disorders, constipation can be an unexpected side effect that often goes unnoticed. Surprisingly, a study found a significant connection between chronic constipation and eating disorders, with 19 per cent of patients experiencing both conditions simultaneously. Binge eating disorder has also been linked to constipation, along with symptoms like bloating and abdominal pain.

When someone eats too little or has irregular eating patterns, it can slow down the body's natural digestion process. The body adapts by conserving energy and resources, which, while impressive, can increase the risk of constipation. This adds another layer of complexity to the already challenging journey of healing and recovery. Other contributing factors may include dehydration, electrolyte imbalances, psychological stress, and, in some cases, laxative abuse.

Dealing with an eating disorder is a deeply personal and tough journey. If you or someone you know is facing these issues, please understand that you're not alone, and support is available. Addressing the underlying causes, seeking professional guidance and approaching the body's needs with compassion can pave the way for a healthier and more balanced life.

Fluctuations in female sex hormones

Female hormones such as oestrogen and progesterone have quite an impact on your gut. Oestrogen is a constipation friend, as it actually helps keep things moving smoothly in your digestive system. On the flip side, progesterone is a bit of a relaxed character. It tends to calm down the smooth muscles in your intestines, which can slow down waste transit and lead to constipation. You might notice this more during the weeks leading up to your period when progesterone levels are higher, or maybe with hormonal changes in perimenopause and menopause too.

Pregnancy can also bring on constipation, especially in the later stages. As the uterus expands, it puts pressure on your intestines. Plus, those hormonal shifts during pregnancy can lead to reduced intestinal muscle tone, less physical activity and dietary changes – all factors that contribute to constipation.

Your gut microbiome isn't just hanging around, minding its own business. It's actually quite involved in the world of hormones, especially oestrogen, one of the key players. Scientists have come up with a fun new name for this relationship – they call it the 'microgenderome'. This partnership is a two-way street. Hormones can chat with your gut microbiome, and the microbiome can chat right back. They influence each other's actions. So your gut and hormones have this fascinating and intricate relationship going on. We can look forward to knowing more about this in the years to come.

Psychological factors

Stress and tension can help tip the scales of our body's internal balancing act. Imagine a tug-of-war between our stress responses ('fight or flight') and our relaxation response ('rest and digest'). When the balance is off, it can throw our digestive system into a bit of a loop, potentially making things move more sluggishly and leading to constipation.

A link has been found between constipation and certain personality traits, including avoidance, obsession and even narcissism. When analysing stress-coping methods, one group of researchers identified two main approaches: 'monitoring' (where individuals overthink potential issues) and 'blunting' (where they avoid stressors). Interestingly, those using the 'blunting' approach had more constipation issues. Constipated individuals also seem to have heightened anxiety and perfectionist tendencies, although there is still nothing definitively known about these associations.

Experiencing constipation can sometimes be also linked to challenging life experiences. Events such as bereavement, job loss, moving homes, major illnesses or surgeries, relationship issues and divorce, financial problems, childbirth, and experience of trauma can leave an unexpected mark on our health, including our digestion. When we face difficulties like these, our body switches into the 'fight or flight' mode and prioritises immediate survival. Unfortunately, this can mean that our regular, everyday processes, including digestion, take a back seat. This shift can lead to a slowdown in our digestive system and, for some of us, this might result in constipation. Intriguingly, women who've endured depression, anxiety or trauma, or who suffer from post-traumatic stress disorder (PTSD) and tend to withdraw from life, are more susceptible to constipation. It's a case of feeling stuck in your life and, as a result, being stuck in your bowel.

Physical abuse can place our bodies in a constant state of stress, potentially leading to disruptions in bowel movements. Neglect, especially during childhood, may result in prolonged stress, affecting psychological well-being. The profound and deeply personal consequences of sexual abuse reach far beyond the immediate emotional and psychological scars, often manifesting in ways one might not immediately connect to the traumatic event. In a study examining the connection between digestive disorders and past experiences, a significant finding emerged. A staggering 40 per cent of individuals with lower functional digestive issues (for example, constipation) reported having been victims of sexual abuse.

It's not just physical issues we're dealing with. The emotional fallout from stress or trauma, like anxiety and depression, often manifests physically, sometimes as a condition like constipation. This is closely linked to our gut–brain axis, the vital communication channel that connects our emotional and mental health with our digestive system. Additionally, in coping with these traumatic experiences, our eating habits might shift, often gravitating towards comfort foods that may be less nutritious. And, for those who might be on medications to manage post-traumatic symptoms, constipation can emerge as an unexpected side effect. It's vital to approach this with compassion and gentle understanding, recognising that the body and mind have intricate ways of coping. Knowing this connection is part of the broader picture of healing and self-understanding. Remember, you're not alone on this journey, and understanding these links might just be another step towards holistic well-being.

So it appears that stress, early life experiences, trauma and even personality traits may all influence constipation. To truly grasp constipation's narrative, we need to zoom out and view the mind and body as one. This underscores the importance of creating dedicated space for relaxation and confidence to seek additional support if needed.

If you have been, or are, going through a period of trauma, anxiety, frustration, feeling trapped – and your digestive system is off – it may be that these psychological factors are being mirrored in your digestive distress. It's okay to reach out to a trusted friend or family member and open up about your feelings. Seeking guidance from a counsellor or therapist can also be a valuable step to consider. You deserve understanding, support and to heal during these tough moments, and it's okay to seek help and prioritise your well-being.

Obsession with bowels and psychological distress

It's true that some individuals may find themselves thinking a lot about various aspects of their bathroom habits, such as the regularity, appearance and consistency of their stools, as well as the satisfaction of bowel movements or the feeling of incomplete evacuation afterwards. Depending on the severity and impact on daily life, this can be categorised as an obsessive-compulsive disorder (OCD) or another related condition. Some experts say it may even be more common that we realise. People with these behaviours may spend a significant amount of time examining their bowel movements or keeping records of them. While it's okay to pay attention to our digestion, becoming overly focused on it can lead to unnecessary stress and impact daily life.

Research has explored the connection between constipation and OCD. Interestingly, a clear link wasn't found in men, but women showed a connection between OCD and constipation. Some individuals with OCD, for example, may become excessively concerned about cleanliness, even in their daily bathroom habits. They might feel a strong urge to ensure complete bowel emptying, sometimes using products to achieve this goal. This overlap between OCD and bowel habits underscores the close relationship between physical health and mental well-being.

Travel-related constipation

Constipation related to travel is a common problem that affects so many people, including those who usually have no issues with regular bowel movements! It's as if, while you're setting off on a trip, your bowel decides to follow its own itinerary – one where it slows down and misbehaves.

Travelling long distances, particularly when crossing multiple time zones, is something your bowel might protest about. One common trend is how our body's routines, including mealtimes and sleep, get disrupted during travelling. This shift can throw off our body's internal clock, making bowel movements less predictable. In some cases, even short-distance travel can affect the sensitive and complex nature of the digestive system. Then there are the prolonged periods of sitting during long flights or road trips, which may affect the bowel's functioning.

Air travel presents its own unique challenges. The pressure changes in airplane cabins can lead to bloating and discomfort, and the thought of navigating the cramped airplane toilet can be daunting. When back on the ground, unfamiliar or questionably clean public toilets can deter us from timely relief. Plus, with the inherent stresses of modern travel – from catching flights to securing accommodation – our digestion can go further awry.

While trying out diverse foods and eating out are major highlights for many, sudden dietary shifts, particularly those lacking in fibre, can leave us feeling backed up. Combine this with the dehydration from long days, hot climates or booze, and our digestion can truly feel the strain. The remedy will be unique to you – discover what suits you best from the wide array of dietary solutions, eating habits, supplements and laxatives discussed in the upcoming pages.

Conclusion

There's no doubt that constipation is a complex condition. Its many forms can be bewildering as they do not always have clear-cut causes, but they can be linked to a wide range of processes and potential triggers. Also, every individual's experience with constipation is unique, shaped by a myriad of personal factors. The scientific journey to fully understanding and effectively treating it continues.

Given its impact not just on our health and well-being, but also on our pockets, it's all the more crucial to stay informed and seek the best solutions. But what's reassuring is that, with a holistic approach and understanding, you can begin to see the bigger picture and the best solution(s). If constipation is weighing you down, remember it's not just about what you've eaten or how much you've moved – it's about understanding YOU. And if things get tough, seeking expert guidance can help put the pieces together, offering the support and solutions tailored just for you.

•CHAPTER 4•

THE MICROBIOME

In 1935, the first president of the British Society of Gastroenterology, Sir Arthur Hurst, declared, 'No organ in the body is as misunderstood, maligned and inadequately addressed as the colon.' Only now, nine decades later, are we finally beginning to appreciate the complexities of the gut – how its work involves so much more than absorbing nutrients and eliminating waste. We are in an era where this once overlooked organ is recognised as crucial to our overall health and well-being, with particular focus on the microbiome – the collection of trillions of tiny organisms that reside there.

Your microbiome is a lively society of somewhere to the effect of around 40 *trillion* microbial residents (that's 40,000,000,000,000), with most living in your large intestine. And while this is not an exact count, it highlights the immense scale of the microbial communities inside of us. These microbes are predominantly bacteria, spanning roughly 1,000 distinct bacterial species, but also include fungi, protozoa, Archaea and viruses. Recent estimates suggest that the number of these microbial inhabitants is roughly the same as the number of human cells in the body – so we're equal parts human and microbe!

Having a wide variety of different microorganisms in your gut promotes gut health. Imagine your gut microbes as a complex ecosystem, with each microbe playing a unique role in maintaining balance. However, the ideal gut microbiome remains a mystery. The diversity and numbers of these different microbes in our gut can be influenced by so many things such as your mode of delivery at birth, how you were fed as a baby, age, gender, diet, hygiene, living environment, health conditions, medications, and even where you live. From the moment we're born, our gut starts to be populated by these microbes.

The community of microbes, collectively referred to as the 'microbiota', exists in two states. The first is a balanced state, termed 'eubiosis', where the microbes remain stable. A balanced gut microbiota composition is essential for the optimal operation of other body organs. The second state is an imbalance, referred to as 'dysbiosis', which can occur as a result of various factors, including the rapid increase of specific types of bacteria, the invasion of pathogenic bacteria, the use of antibiotics, or significant changes in diet. This imbalance can lead to an overgrowth of potentially harmful microbes, known as pathogens, which then have the opportunity to outcompete the beneficial ones. An imbalance can also activate the immune system in ways that promote inflammation in the gut. Dysbiosis has been linked to various health issues, with constipation and IBS part of the fallout.

Gut microbiome 101

These tiny inhabitants in your colon are quite diverse and can be examined through stool analysis. Interestingly, what you eat plays a significant role in this microbial diversity, accounting for about 57 per cent of the variation in your gut microbiota. Genetic differences, on the other hand, contribute only 12 per cent. Changing your diet, such as transitioning from a typical Western diet high in fats and low in fibre to one that's more plant-based and fibre-rich, can rapidly alter the composition of these gut microorganisms, sometimes in as little as 24 hours.

You've also got little bugs that call the mucosal lining of your gut home. This lining is like a protective layer of mucus along your digestive tract. They play a crucial role in how your gut communicates with the tissue just beneath its lining. This includes influencing the immune response and the activities of cells that release hormones in the gut, which, in the grand scheme of things, can also impact digestion. Research has consistently shown that these tiny organisms living in our gut have a mutually beneficial relationship with us humans – we are the best of friends, until that is, there's a disagreement.

Your gut bugs' job description

These microbial residents have an insanely busy job, and perhaps the most interesting job in the world. They train and support our immune responses and influence how the cells lining our intestines behave and function. They also like to gossip with our brain, influencing our mood and mental functions. Not only do they lend a hand in producing vital vitamins, but they also act as a defence mechanism, warding off harmful bacteria invading our gut. They are far from being just passive dwellers; rather, they interact deeply with all our bodily systems.

They also break down the stuff in your food that your body can't digest and produce essential short-chain fatty acids (SCFAs). SCFAs play a vital role in keeping your gut healthy. They are made when your body ferments dietary fibre in the large intestine, and the main ones to know are acetate, propionate and butyrate. They're primarily produced in the first part of your large intestine. More importantly, research has even shown that when SCFA levels in your stools go up, constipation symptoms tend to go down.

The constipation ecosystem

Think of the gut microbiota as a delicate living system. When something disrupts this balance, it can set off a chain reaction in our bodies, and constipation might be one of the potential outcomes. It's notable that an imbalance – or dysbiosis – of gut microbes has been observed in individuals experiencing constipation. What remains to be clarified is whether this microbial imbalance is a *result* of constipation or a direct *cause*.

One interesting trail has led to researchers looking at Archaea. These are microorganisms capable of surviving in Earth's most extreme environments, like hot springs, deep-sea vents and highly acidic waters. They have also been found in our digestive system and appear to have a unique talent – they can produce methane. This could be a problem, as scientists have observed that higher levels of methane in the gut are linked to firmer stools and constipation. It's like methane has the power to slow down the food's journey through the intestines.

Inconsistencies in nailing down the constipation–microbe connection arise as a result of factors such as diet, age, psychological distress and health status, along with environment, location, lifestyle and habits – each of which can play a significant role in shaping and influencing gut microbe levels and composition. Finding needles in haystacks comes to mind! So, although microbe involvement is certainly real, there's just still so much to learn.

In summary, a better understanding of the gut microbiota's intricate role in constipation could lead the way to targeting specific microbial interactions and pathways and discovering more effective remedies to ensure bowel issues are better managed.

The gut–brain axis

When talking about the microbiome, we also need to mention the gut–brain axis. Picture a two-way communication superhighway that bridges your digestive system and your brain. It is both fascinating and enigmatic. When we examine conditions like constipation and IBS-C, the gut–brain axis emerges as a previously underrated player. The relationship resembles an intimate partnership involving both the gut and the brain. Here are some of the interesting connections at play:

- *Emotions and stress:* The brain wields a significant influence over the gut. Various emotional states, including stress, anxiety and excitement, have the power to send signals to the digestive system, thereby impacting its functionality. In times of stress, for instance, the gut might respond by slowing its processes, increasing the risk of constipation.

- *Gut microbiota:* These beneficial microbes are capable of producing compounds that communicate with the brain. An imbalance in the gut's microbial population can disrupt the production of these beneficial compounds, potentially triggering shifts in bowel habits, affecting regularity and comfort.

- *Pain and discomfort:* Both constipation and IBS-C are often accompanied by abdominal discomfort or pain. These sensations can relay messages to the brain, heightening the individual's awareness of their gut issues and potentially aggravating the condition.

Understanding the nuances of the gut–brain axis plays a part in the process for managing constipation and IBS-C. By tackling stress and nurturing a healthy gut microbiome, you can help to positively influence this delicate and complex connection, paving the way for improved digestive health and overall well-being. More on this later (see Chapter 13).

Gut speed

Do you recall that the speed at which food moves through our gut – or 'gut transit time' – can vary not just from one person to another but also within the same person from day to day? Well, it appears that this change in speed can impact things like the number and type of microbes in our gut. But our microbes can also impact rate of motility, creating a two-way relationship. And the speed can impact how our diet interacts with the microbes present. In a nutshell, the way your poo looks has a strong connection to the types of bacteria in your gut. But there's a long way to go to understanding this fully.

Serotonin, bile acids and gut motility

When discussing constipation, it's crucial to also mention the role of the neurotransmitter serotonin. Often recognised for its impact on mood and brain function, serotonin is primarily produced in the gut. In fact, about 90 to 95 per cent of the body's total serotonin is synthesised and released by cells in the gut known as enterochromaffin cells. Serotonin is pivotal in maintaining the smooth operation of the digestive system, overseeing processes such as the movement of food and enzyme activity, and influencing gut sensitivity. Moreover, serotonin communicates with the brain via the gut–brain axis, and this communication pathway plays a vital role in influencing both digestive well-being and mental health.

Further deepening this close relationship is the connection between our gut microbiota and the body's serotonin system. The diverse microorganisms residing in our gut have the capacity to influence the production and release of serotonin, directly impacting gut health.

Additionally, our gut microbiota plays a role in modulating bile acids. These bile acids, essential for digestion, can vary in type and amount based on the microbial composition of the gut. This variation can significantly influence gut motility, which is particularly relevant in the context of constipation. By affecting the movement of the digestive tract, these modified bile acids can either alleviate or worsen constipation. In these complex connections in our gut, every step, twist and turn matters in helping us capture a holistic picture of our inner ecosystem and gut workings; even if we don't yet fully understand all the specifics, but know they are involved.

Diet and gut interactions

Plant-based foods have the admirable role of feeding your gut microbes. When the microbes in our gut ferment these fibres, they create something like a magnetic pull that draws water into the bowel. This process is believed to speed up the journey of food through our intestines. When fibre undergoes fermentation, it's thought to also contribute to forming bulkier stools, again as a result of the production of SCFAs, which are linked to boosting colonic motility. These SCFAs also support a diverse population of gut bacteria.

It's really important to keep our gut microbes happy by feeding them the right stuff. If we don't give them enough fibre and other nutrients such as those found in plant-based foods, they might start munching on proteins from our diet, or even nibble on our gut lining – which you don't want to happen. You see, when they break down fibre, it's usually a good thing – think of the SCFAs. But when they start digesting proteins, it can lead to some not-so-friendly by-products, like branched-chain fatty acids (BCFAs), phenols and certain gases, which may have a less-than-desirable impact on our health.

It's not ideal if our gut microbes begin to use the mucous lining of our gut as a food source, because the mucous lining is the protective barrier for our intestines, preventing harmful substances like bacteria and irritants from damaging the delicate tissues underneath. If the microbes become mischievous in their search for nutrients and start breaking this lining down – which has been shown in animal studies – this can lead to a weaker gut barrier, potentially making way for various gut issues, and maybe impacting constipation, maybe not. But why take the chance? So it's super important to keep those gut bugs well fed with a fibre-rich diet to avoid them turning to protein or our gut lining for snacks.

Lastly, it's worth mentioning that the fermentation of fibre in the gut can lead to the production of gas, which might result in discomfort such as bloating or excessive farting for some people. To be more specific, some foods may cause increased gas in some individuals! Finding the right balance in fibre intake is crucial for managing constipation effectively. And this, ladies and gentlemen, is a commitment that pays off. For tips on how to achieve this balance, turn to this book's treatment of fibre in Chapters 6 to 9, where we explore strategies for increasing fibre intake without the discomfort.

Thirty plants per week keeps your gut unique: a quest for microbial diversity

The American Gut Project stands as one of the most extensive and comprehensive science initiatives exploring the human microbiome. The researchers behind this work have been exploring how various factors such as diet, lifestyle and even the types of medications we take can influence the make-up of our gut microbiome. They've observed that individuals who eat a wide variety of plant-based foods – we're talking 30 different types each week – tend to have a more diverse microbiome. Why is this diversity a good thing? Picture your gut with its vibrant ecosystem, where every microbe has its own special job. Some are great at breaking down vegetables, while others excel at making certain vitamins or supporting our immune system. The more diverse this community is, the more resilient and effective it can be at keeping everything in balance and keeping you healthy. A diverse gut microbiome is also associated with improved digestion. So, by getting all those different plant-based foods into your diet – fruits, veg, wholegrains, nuts, seeds, legumes, and even herbs and spices– you're essentially going to be able to better feed all your microbes to help keep them thriving.

In your journey to enrich the diversity of plant-based foods in your diet, a great strategy is to embrace variety and visualise yourself exploring every aisle of the supermarket, hopefully enthusiastically adding a wide array of foods from different groups into your trolley! Each shopping trip can be an opportunity to discover a new vegetable or fruit you haven't tried before. For example, embracing seasonal and local produce can add an element of freshness and sustainability to your culinary journey. Seasonal fruits and vegetables are often at their peak in flavour and nutrients, and choosing local produce supports your community and reduces your carbon footprint. Don't forget about fermented veg either. Items like sauerkraut and kimchi are excellent choices that can introduce beneficial microbes into your gut ecosystem.

You might also consider exploring different grains and legumes. Each type of grain – such as oats, quinoa, barley or buckwheat – brings its own unique flavour and texture to your meals, along with a host of nutrients and fibres that are great for your gut. Legumes such as lentils, chickpeas and various beans are also fantastic fibre-rich additions to your diet. Experimenting with herbs and spices, either fresh or dried, is another gut-healthy way to diversify your meals. By adding these elements to your diet, you not only make each meal more interesting and enjoyable, but also do something of great benefit to your gut health.

To gauge your progress in maintaining overall gut health, consider maintaining a food log like the one provided here. Take some time to jot down all the fibre-rich foods you consume. Achieving a count of 30 different plant-based foods over the week is a great indicator that you're on the right track for optimal gut health.

As you look at the results of your food log, noting each fibre-rich and plant-based food you consume, consider this exercise as a seamless segue into the next chapters. There, the diet side of managing constipation will unfold before your eyes, offering a deeper and more detailed understanding. So, keep your diversity log – it can be an eye-opener – and get ready for an exciting journey through the dietary landscape in upcoming chapters!

My fibre log

Fruit	Vegetables	Wholegrains	Beans and pulses	Nuts and seeds

How to interpret your fibre log

The goal isn't to obsess over reaching an exact 30 types of plant-based foods. Instead it's about seeing where you're at so you can get a feel for how diverse your diet is over a week when you add up all the different foods in each of the categories. If you have 10 per week, try to increase to 15, then to 20 over time. It's more beneficial to focus on broadening and varying your diet rather than fixating on achieving a perfect 30 every single week.

•CHAPTER 5•
MY CONSTIPATION PROFILE

Undesirable changes in your bowel habits, such as constipation along with gut symptoms like bloating, gas and pain, can be incredibly debilitating, exhausting and socially isolating. These symptoms are highly individual and can evolve over time, making it challenging to find effective solutions. What may have worked for someone else might not have the same impact on you. However, this section is designed exclusively for you. You'll be led through the journey of understanding your constipation and gut symptoms by identifying patterns that are simple to track.

Gaining insight is the essential first step in empowering yourself to overcome the limitations of gut discomfort. As you monitor different elements that might influence and trigger your symptoms, you'll cultivate a deep understanding of the connection between your gut and your constipation. Although there are many apps available, using an old-school pen to paper technique can be an effective method to actively engage with your body and its habits. The act of writing stimulates both analytical and creative thinking, sharpening your focus and prompting you to observe and link patterns.

In our quest for a normal life, many aspects of our day-to-day living run on autopilot. But ongoing gut issues are a sign that something is amiss. These symptoms can sap your physical and mental energy, and impact your sleep, mood and *joie de vivre*. This part of the book invites you to examine both what you write down and what you reflect on. Adopting this approach empowers you to identify what might be going on in your life that is making constipation hang around too long.

The process serves as a tool to empower you with a deeper understanding of what's going on. Still, it's essential to consult with your GP if you're experiencing gut issues such as changes in bowel habits, abdominal pain or bloating.

My constipation story

Organise and explain your constipation experiences using the following prompts.

1. I have been constipated since

2. Medical tests and investigations

3. My medical team

4. Family and friends that support me

5. Constipation affects me by

6. This helps my constipation

7. This doesn't help

8. I am grateful for

These obstacles get in my way of reaching my goals – for example, making changes to my diet, exercising, relaxing, getting enough sleep.

My baseline symptom profile

Bristol stool form scale			Tick relevant box(es)	Bowel frequency	Tick relevant box(es)
Type 1 Severe constipation		Separate hard lumps, hard to pass		Less than once a week	
Type 2 Mild constipation		Sausage-shape, but lumpy		Once every 4–6 days	
Type 3 Normal		Like a sausage, but with cracks on its surface		Once every 2–3 days	
				Once a day	
Type 4 Normal		Like a sausage or snake, smooth and soft		2–3 times per day	ı ı
Type 5 Lacking fibre		Soft blobs with clear-cut edges		4–6 times per day	
Type 6 Mild diarrhoea		Fluffy pieces, mushy stool		>7 times per day	
Type 7 Severe diarrhoea		No solid pieces, entirely liquid		My bowel frequency is erratic!	ı

Symptoms (in the last 2 weeks)	Rate from 1 to 4 (1 = none, 4 = severe)	Symptoms (in the last 2 weeks)	Rate from 1 to 4 (1 = none, 4 = severe)
Bloating		Poor appetite	
Wind or gas		Nausea	
Abdominal pain		Tiredness	
Incomplete evacuation*		Headaches	
Belching or burping		Brain fog	
Reflux		Anxiety or depression	

*A feeling of not being able to complete a bowel movement.

Habit tracker

Embarking on a journey to manage constipation often requires making meaningful lifestyle changes. But how can you ensure you stick to these changes and turn them into habits that last? Enter the Habit Tracker – your trusty companion on the road to sustained diet and lifestyle changes. From daily fibre intake and hydration goals to regular exercise and stress management, the Habit Tracker provides a structured way to implement positive changes.

Identify what you want to change or make happen in your life. It doesn't have to be 20 things. Just one or two can be enough. By visually tracking your progress and celebrating each successful day, you'll find motivation and accountability. Whether you're working with a healthcare provider or taking charge of your gut health independently, the Habit Tracker is a great way to build habits that lead to lasting relief from constipation. Start tracking; start to help you (and your microbes) thrive.

Habit Tracker

Examples of habits / Your turn	Break the fast	H_2O	2 max coffees	Daylight walk	Breeeeathe!	Meet Emma	CHEW, CHEW, CHEW	Psyllium husks	Bed by 11 o'clock	Toilet tricks	Probiotic	Eat the rainbow	Grow herbs	Phone Ma	New recipes	Culture night	2-3 fruits	Pack lunch	Read a chapter
1																			
2																			
3																			
4																			
5																			
6																			
7																			
8																			
9																			
10																			
11																			
12																			
13																			
14																			
15																			
16																			
17																			
18																			
19																			
20																			
21																			
22																			
23																			
24																			
25																			
26																			
27																			
28																			
29																			
30																			

Mark each box with a symbol '✗' or '✓' or colour code ... whatever you find most pleasing.

Habit tracker

This tracker creates a visual cue to remind you to do your thing, and it motivates you, as you can see the progress you are making. It also feels satisfying to record your success in the moment!

Success comes from what you do consistently!

Food, lifestyle, mind and gut diary

Journalling in the suggested format here aims to make *you* the constipation detective untangling the mystery of your gut. You can get the most out of your diary by using these prompts below. Plus, you get to figure out what works best for you, whether you're flying solo or getting support from a dietitian. Daily prompts help you record factors like food, fluids and eating behaviours. It's not just about food and eating, though! Your journal will cover everything from how you're feeling – your sleep patterns, exercise, stress levels – to how even your menstrual cycle might be affecting you (for females), along with notes on any supplements or medications you're taking. All of this adds up to some really valuable insights about your body.

You can visit www.guthealthmatters.ie and download a free two-week diary. Use the code WYCG24.

Prompts to get the most out of your journalling

Diet

- Make an effort to record everything you eat and drink throughout the day, including between-meal snacks. Consistency will provide a more accurate picture of your eating habits.

- Consider how your food is prepared (freshly cooked or reheated) and the cooking methods used.

- Reflect on portion sizes (small, medium or large).

- How often do you eat out or rely on takeaway or prepackaged meals versus cooking from scratch at home?

- Observe how many high-fat and high-sugar foods are in your diet. Are there too many?

- Note the number of high-fibre foods you include at meals and snacks. Can this be improved?

- Note the consumption of any protein supplements, chewing gum and sugar-free foods, which can sometimes increase gut symptoms such as bloating and gas.

- Reflect on the variety of your diet, including all food groups. Are you avoiding a full food group like dairy or grains?

- Observe your fluid intake and any connections between caffeine, carbonated drinks, juice, alcohol, and your bowel habit and gut symptoms.

- Do you add salt to your food?

Bowel movements and gut symptoms
- Track the frequency of your bowel movements and their nature (type, any difficulty, completeness).

- Note any abdominal pain before and after bowel movements and its pattern.

- Observe your main symptoms (pain, bloating, gas, tiredness) and their timing (morning or evening).

Eating behaviour
- Consider your chewing habits and meal duration.

- Evaluate the regularity of your mealtimes and any tendencies to skip meals.

- Observe if you graze on food throughout the day or eat a lot at night.

- Reflect on how you feel emotionally while eating. Do you have any anxiety related to food?

- Explore whether thoughts of food dominate your life. If you find that they do, remember that seeking support and guidance is always an option.

Lifestyle factors

- Record the use of medication, probiotics and any supplements you take for managing constipation and gut symptoms. Do they help?

- Monitor stress levels and emotions to help identify their effects on your gut.

- For females, consider menstrual cycle patterns and their influence on your bowel and symptoms, if any.

- Are you active day to day? Try to incorporate regular exercise – a combination of aerobic and strength-based exercise is a good idea.

- Prioritise quality sleep – seven to nine hours of uninterrupted sleep is optimal.

- Do you make time to relax? Practices like deep belly breathing, yoga, meditation, or walks in the fresh air are excellent ways to relax.

Reflections and 'aha' moments

- Use this space to reflect on positive aspects of your day, such as moments of gratitude, enjoyment, improvement or happiness.

- Celebrate the good days. Also reflect on challenging days, providing structure to your feelings and helping you process them.

Celebrate every gain!

- Record your achievements and newly formed habits.

- Your diary serves as a progress log, offering insights into how far you've come since you began this journey.

- Stay honest and true in your journal, knowing it's a tool for self-care and self-improvement, free from judgement.

- Keep it private to create a safe space for personal expression.

- Your diary signifies your commitment to self-care and self-improvement. Grab your pen and embark on your gut-symptom-unravelling project. And best of luck on your journey!

Who should keep a diary?

The ideal moment to commence this diary is right now, and it's advisable to maintain it for as long as it proves beneficial, with a recommended duration of two weeks. You can then enhance your understanding by repeating the process from time to time, but especially if things are not going according to plan.

Please keep in mind that if the diary ever feels like a chore, if it's incomplete, or especially if it elevates stress levels, or leads to an unhealthy fixation on food, it's perfectly fine to take a break or not to continue at all. Your well-being is paramount, and this diary is meant to be a tool for self-improvement and understanding, not a source of added stress.

Sample food and symptom diary – part 1

Day: _____ Date: _____

Dietary factors	Food	Bowel movements and gut symptoms
Breakfast		
AM snack		
Lunch		
PM snack		
Dinner		
Bedtime snack		

Fluids		
Water	O O O O O O O O	Comments
Coffee/tea	O O O O O O O O	
Other drinks	O O O O O O O O	
Alcohol	O O O O O O O O	

Sample food and symptom diary – part 2

Eating behaviour			
Rate of eating	O Slow	O Moderate	O Fast
Chewing food until pulp-like	O Yes	O No	
Regular meals	O Breakfast	O Lunch	O Dinner
Food anxiety level	O Low	O Moderate	O High

Lifestyle factors

Medications	Probiotics/supplements
Stress and emotions	Menstrual status

Exercise	Type(s) .... Duration ....
Sleep	Went to bed at: .... Got up at:.............................. Slept soundly or tossed and turned? .... Feel energised or feel like staying in bed? ....
Relaxation time	Type(s) .... Duration ....

Today's reflections	Today's 'aha' moment

This comprehensive exploration aims to empower you to better understand your gut's unique responses and needs, ultimately guiding you towards improvement with your constipation and your overall digestive health and well-being. Remember that this journal is your personal tool, tailored to your life and symptoms. Your journey is unique, and your progress should be measured against your own experiences and goals.

Time to review progress

When you maintain your diary for up to two weeks, it will provide you with valuable insights into your experience with constipation. To guide your reflection on your current state of affairs and future goals, consider completing this exercise with the prompts provided below.

Time to review progress!

My feelings about my condition:

- O _____
- O _____
- O _____
- O _____
- O _____
- O _____

My main challenges are:

- O _____
- O _____
- O _____
- O _____
- O _____
- O _____

Strategies I find helpful for constipation:

- O _____
- O _____
- O _____
- O _____
- O _____
- O _____

What I have learned in the past 2 weeks:

- O _____
- O _____
- O _____
- O _____
- O _____
- O _____

Things that make my constipation and symptoms worse:

- O _____
- O _____
- O _____
- O _____
- O _____
- O _____

Goals for the next 2 weeks:

- O _____
- O _____
- O _____
- O _____
- O _____
- O _____

My support team:

- O _____
- O _____
- O _____
- O _____
- O _____
- O _____

How I will implement these goals:

- O _____
- O _____
- O _____
- O _____
- O _____
- O _____

•CHAPTER 6•

DIET

We've all heard the age-old advice: to alleviate constipation woes, simply increase your intake of fibre and fluids. This can actually work for many, which is brilliant. Keep it going! But if you've done that and it hasn't worked, you'll know how frustrating that advice is. As with numerous health guidelines, delving deeper often uncovers a reality that is much more nuanced.

So let's clear the air right from the start: there isn't a universal diet or constipation remedy that fits everyone's needs. Discovering the right solution is a personal journey. It's about understanding your body's unique needs and responses, and then tailoring a plan that works specifically for you. In the pages ahead, you'll find a wealth of different strategies and approaches to guide you in finding the dietary solution that suits you best.

How well these dietary changes work really depends on a variety of factors, including how much fibre and the types of fibre you consume, the type of constipation and gut symptoms you have, and broader lifestyle factors – your activity and stress levels, for example. So, does increasing fibre and fluid intake truly work? The best answer is that 'probably, but it depends!'

Dietary goals

In addressing chronic constipation, the goal needs to extend beyond having more bowel motions every week. It should include the aspiration for a seamless and pain-free poo, unimpeded by any exit barriers and devoid of discomfort and bloating. You want your poo to be just right – not too hard, not too soft – and to feel like you've got it all out.

The selection and sequence of treatments are going to be better when you plot yourself on the 'constipation wheel' (you can do that next) and decide on the best starting point. If you're ready to make dietary adjustments, know that it will involve a bit of trial and error as you discover what foods work best for your body.

Constipation wheel

When it comes to managing constipation, your initial steps should involve adjustments to your diet and lifestyle. However, if you're already following a high-fibre diet and experiencing infrequent bowel movements that are hard and incomplete, it's going to be more effective to first focus on 'clearing out' what is backed up in there first. This can often mean using rescue laxatives, so have a chat with your GP about the best choice for you.

If you start to load up on fibre and nothing happens except that it brings on symptoms like bloating, stomach pain and gas, it's time to pull back and try to get things moving another way. No one needs that extra discomfort. If you have tried fibre and laxatives and you've had limited success, it's time to investigate your pelvic floor.

Visualise this. Your poo, stuck in your bowel, is a large jumbo jet sitting idly on the runway. Just like a jumbo jet preparing for take-off (or a flush down the toilet), it requires a specific level of force and thrust. Essentially, the engines need to rev up. In cases of constipation, the typical engine power, represented by the usual advice of increasing dietary fibre and water, might not suffice to get the necessary 'clearance'. This is where the concept of boosting engine power using specific fibres and/or laxatives comes into play. Once the jumbo jet is airborne and cruising, you can gradually reduce the engine's acceleration (that is, the use of laxatives), allowing other fuel sources, such as fibre and fluid, to operate more efficiently.

Alternatively, consider a scenario where the jumbo jet boasts optimal engine power, yet is unable to take off because of a technical malfunction (in the case of constipation, this could be attributed to pelvic floor dysfunction). Regardless of how much acceleration (fibre, water or laxatives) you have at your disposal, take-off remains elusive, potentially worsening constipation. In this case, the only effective approach to address the malfunction (pelvic floor dysfunction) is to seek assistance from the aircraft maintenance technicians, or in this context, a pelvic health physiotherapist.

1. Assess your profile

2. Implement diet, lifestyle, supplement/probiotic advice

3. If 'stuck', clear with medication*

4. If diet, lifestyle and medications are unhelpful, request pelvic floor examination

*request GP assessment

As you progress through the solutions offered in this book, keep these scenarios in mind. Whether you're dealing with a stationary jumbo jet or addressing a technical fault, every section of this part of the book is designed to ensure your 'jumbo' (poo) continues its regular flights and arrives on schedule (ranging from three times a day to once every one to three days) throughout its lifespan.

The role of diet in relieving constipation

In your constipation toolkit, consider dietary control to be your reliable first line of defence. However, most people know this when they face the challenges of constipation, with or without IBS. Most have probably tried increasing fibre. They've loaded up on all the usual suspects, from oats to seeds to beans, waiting for the magic to happen. They diligently bring the water bottle with them and top it up regularly throughout the day. All of this takes commitment and planning. So when there's no improvement, they can feel very discouraged and at their wits' end. It's completely understandable.

For others, the dietary road can get even bumpier at this point, especially if other gut symptoms like abdominal pain or discomfort, bloating and gas are lurking around. They might start to question every food choice, wondering if there's some hidden intolerance throwing their system off balance. They start to cut out foods like wheat, dairy and coffee and yet still suffer. It can feel like just fumbling in the dark trying to find the culprit that's keeping them stuck. It's easy to fail in the constipation dietary test or to consider restricting your diet bit by bit. It can also lead to increased anxiety around eating. But rest assured, you haven't really done a whole pile wrong – the issue is that one-size-fits-all advice simply doesn't cut it. And here's the thing: when it comes to fibres, not all of them are created equal. All fibres are useful, but some fibres prove to be more useful than others. When science leads the way, it will be easier to see the light at the end of the colon!

Fibre SOS

It's time to make peace with your fibre friends. Did you know that as humans our digestive system doesn't break down fibre, like it does protein, fat and starch? Instead, fibre cruises through our digestive system untouched until it hits the colon or large intestine. In the colon, it's greeted by those trillions of microbes mentioned earlier. Fibre serves as *their* primary source of energy.

The official fibre definition is that 'it consists of all nondigestible carbohydrates that are neither digested nor absorbed in the small intestine'. This means that fibre refers to the parts of plant-based foods – mostly grains, fruit, veg, nuts, seeds, pulses – that are leftovers from human digestion. Fibre foods have a structure made up of three or more linked sugar units, making them not sugar. But wait, there's more. For example, fibre includes substances (such as lignin) that aren't carbohydrates but still play a part in the fibre structures. There are also resistant starches, whose make-up shields them from digestive enzymes, meaning they resist digestion.

Constipation aside, fibre is a champion for your general health. For example, it keeps you full, which can help in maintaining a healthy weight. It manages your blood sugar, which is excellent for helping reduce diabetes risk. It can reduce bad cholesterol for a happy heart, and by feeding your gut bugs, it can help keep the balance of microbes in the gut in check (and you're now up to speed on what your gut bugs do – for example, helping to keep the protective lining in your gut healthy, serving as a first line of defence against pathogens, influencing the body's inflammatory responses). Fibre is a *must-have*!

Despite these advantages, most of us aren't eating enough fibre. The goal? Approximately 30g per day. In Ireland, the average intake is below 20g. So, in terms of constipation (and to reap all the other health benefits), let's view this fibre gap as an opportunity to include more plant-based goodness in our lives. And we're going to be smart about it, with the added benefit of helping alleviate constipation in the process.

Example of low-fibre intake

Meal	Food	Fibre
Breakfast	Cornflakes	0.9
	Milk	0.0
	Banana	1.1
Snack	Latte	0.0
Lunch	Turkey sandwich with white bread	1.7
	Lettuce	0.2
	Tomato	0.3
	Yogurt	0.0
Snack	Crisps	0.9
Evening meal	Grilled fish	0.0
	Carrots	2.2
	Mashed potatoes	2.8
Total		10.1g

Example of high-fibre intake

Meal	Food	Fibre
Breakfast	Porridge	2.3
	Milk	0.0
	Kiwis	5.4
Snack	Almonds	3.3
Lunch	Turkey sandwich with multigrain bread	4.2
	Lettuce	0.2
	Tomato	0.3
	Mixed seed yogurt	1.1
Snack	Apple	1.8
	Peanut butter	1.2
Evening meal	Grilled fish	0.0
	Roasted veg	5.0
	Sweet potato wedges (with skins)	6.7
Total		31.5g

How do I know how much fibre I'm having?

To get a clear picture of your fibre intake – how much you're consuming and when – consider giving these strategies a try:

- *Food diary:* Kick things off by keeping a detailed record of everything you eat (the food and symptom diary in Chapter 5 is ideal for this). This is not just a routine activity; it's a revealing journey into your fibre-intake habits. As suggested, shoot for two weeks for a detailed view, including weekends of course! If you include two to three fibre foods at each meal and one to two for each snack, you're showing your gut a lot of love. If your current fibre intake is below this level, don't worry. The upcoming pages will guide you in navigating how to gradually and easily increase your dietary fibre intake. You don't need to obsessively count grams of fibre in your diet; it's more beneficial to focus on increasing dietary fibre variety.

- *Nutrition labels:* Most of your packaged foods come with a bonus – they will have nutrition labels detailing fibre content per serving. Utilise this knowledge to make informed choices about your fibre intake. A high-fibre intake is considered >6g fibre per 100g.

- *Listen to your body:* Pay attention to your natural feedback system – listen to your body's natural signals and cues. If you're experiencing consistent and smooth bowel movements, you're hitting the fibre mark (providing you're actually including fibre in your diet!). However, if things are a bit off rhythm, it might be a sign to adjust your fibre levels.

- *Professional guidance:* When you're looking for tailored advice, consult a gut health dietitian. They are the experts ready to give you a tailored evaluation and offer additional helpful advice for your fibre intake.

Understanding your fibre intake is a proactive step towards managing constipation effectively, as it will help you find the right balance that works for you and your digestive health.

Other plant-based components

While fibre often grabs the headlines, it's important to also shine a light on the less-celebrated elements in our diet that can significantly aid in alleviating constipation. Compounds such as sorbitol and polyphenols, both also found in various plant-based foods, can also play a role.

Sorbitol, a natural sugar alcohol found in fruits such as prunes and apples, acts as an osmotic agent, drawing water into the colon, which helps to soften stool and encourage bowel movements. Furthermore, since sorbitol is fermented in the large intestine, the resident bacteria get to work, which may lead to positive changes to your microbiota. While this can be helpful for some, for others it may lead to an increase in gas or discomfort. So for those with constipation, sorbitol might be a sweet solution or something to limit, depending on how your body responds to it.

Polyphenols, which are abundant in fruits, vegetables and drinks such as tea and coffee (and even red wine), contribute to the vibrant colours and antioxidant properties of plant-based foods. They can also act as nourishment for your microbes, promoting the growth of beneficial gut bacteria, which may contribute to regular bowel movements.

In the story of fighting constipation, these natural ingredients might be best described as the trusted wingmen to fibre. Adding a mix of these into your diet will benefit your gut health and reinforce fibre's quest to keep constipation at bay.

Fibre and constipation: what does science really say?

For over a century, scientists have been curious about fibre's effects on constipation. Numerous studies have tried to gather insights and decode its relationship with bowel motions. The results reveal mixed outcomes! Some thorough, high-quality reviews (we're talking meta-analysis and systematic reviews) suggest that adding dietary fibre to your meals can help you become more regular, making your trips to the loo a bit smoother. But other studies don't agree. So it looks like the common suggestion to 'increase your fibre' may not be the magic key for everyone when it comes to constipation. However, scientists didn't always home in on the details of different fibre types, opting in most cases to lump all fibre foods together. This broad-brush method doesn't give us the full picture, because it is just that – too broad! This can lead to overgeneralised conclusions that might not hold true for everyone. And as mentioned, not all fibres work in the same way.

Also, here's something mind-blowing. Astonishingly, in studies focused on fibre supplements for constipation relief, 41 per cent of people reported improvements with a placebo fibre supplement, which highlights the mind's powerful role in digestive health. It also makes the results for those taking the fibre supplement more difficult to interpret.

Moreover, we must recognise that each person's digestive system is unique, and the exact benefits can differ from person to person. However, both European and American guidelines, along with clinical judgement and experience, absolutely recommend using fibre in managing constipation. We just need to be cleverer about choosing the right fibre-rich foods and adjusting to suit each individual's gut.

So while we navigate through the existing research with a critical eye, it's also wise to maintain a balanced view of how fibre, as part of a varied diet, contributes to our well-being, and to recognise the interplay between our mindset and physical health. As healthcare professionals, we're eager for more thorough and well-conducted research that can offer clearer insights into the specific roles of different fibres. But … while we wait for these more carefully planned and executed longer-term and large-scale clinical trials, approximately 15 per cent of us are still suffering with constipation. And people need to be able to get their hands on what constitutes the best available evidence now!

A meta-analysis is like combining the results of many studies on constipation and finding an average score for how effective a treatment, like fibre, is overall.

A systematic review is like gathering and summarising all the available information about using fibre for constipation, similar to reading all the reviews about fibre before deciding if it's right for you.

Clinical judgment is really important alongside both of these methods. It lets healthcare experts use their knowledge and experience to understand the results and give advice based on the overall evidence.

The journey through the large intestine

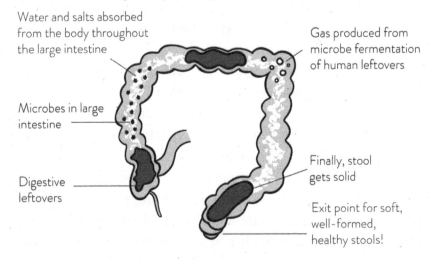

Water and salts absorbed from the body throughout the large intestine

Gas produced from microbe fermentation of human leftovers

Microbes in large intestine

Digestive leftovers

Finally, stool gets solid

Exit point for soft, well-formed, healthy stools!

Imagine the large intestine as a slow-moving conveyor belt. When your digestive leftovers reach the caecum (the beginning of the large intestine), they are typically in liquid form and composed of over 90 per cent water. The trillions of microbes that mostly hang out in the first part, the ascending colon, get stuck in digesting (fermenting) your food leftovers (mainly from plant-based foods). They will release gases in the process, which is important when it comes to deciding which fibre fits into your friend circle.

As the waste moves along the conveyor belt, your body absorbs any remaining water and salts from the semi-digested food. It gets thicker and begins to form what we know as poo. Finally, when the conveyor reaches its end, it's time for it to exit the body. Well-formed stools typically develop in the sigmoid colon and rectum. By the time they reach the rectum (the last section of the large intestine), they will have roughly 75 per cent water content.

And here is something that may surprise you: a typically formed normal stool contains approximately 75 per cent water, a hard stool contains 72 per cent water and a soft stool contains around 77 per cent water. It's incredible how such a tiny tweak in water percentage – thanks to our large intestine's water-absorbing skills – can make a difference between a smooth slide or a stubborn push. Talk about fine margins in the world of poo!

What the f ...

It's okay if you think 'what the fibre is going on', because while fibre is fascinating, it is also complex. You may have heard about the two main types of fibre – soluble and insoluble – but that information is no longer current on its own. Fibre isn't simply split into soluble and insoluble categories. In any case, most foods contain a mix of soluble and insoluble fibre. In the dynamic world of nutrition research, and when looking at which fibre foods help with constipation, we now view fibre based on certain key characteristics that include:

1. **Fermentability:** their ability to be broken down by the gut bacteria

2. **Viscosity:** their ability to thicken or create a gel when they mix with water in the digestive tract

3. **Solubility:** whether they are insoluble or soluble, which refers to their ability to interact with water, which changes depending on how long their chains of sugar molecules are.

So what the f(ibre) do I eat for my stubborn bowel?

Take a bow, soluble, viscous, low-fermented fibres. As they make their way through the large intestine, these fibres are minimally fermented. This helps them hold on to water like a sponge, which increases the chance of keeping your stool soft and easy to pass. This softness is the key to a great bowel movement.

In the world of soluble, viscous fibres that undergo minimal fermentation, psyllium husks stand out the most. Psyllium comes from the husks and seeds of the plant *Plantago ovata*, which is commonly grown in India. Unlike many other fibres, psyllium doesn't ferment in our gut, which means it passes through to the large intestine largely intact, preserving its impressive moisture-retention properties.

Another type of fibre, with the characteristics of insoluble and non-fermentable fibre, is the dietary fibre that does not dissolve in water but is also minimally broken down by the bacteria in the large intestine. Fibre of this type can physically stimulate the lining of our intestines, essentially by promoting water and mucus production, promoting quicker movement and thereby aiding in the swift passage of waste through the bowel. An example of this is coarse wheat bran.

Yet another form of dietary fibre, falling under the category of fermentable fibres, serves as food for your gut microbes, stimulating an increase in poo volume or bulk. This is thought to also increase transit through the bowel. But get this, increased stool volume without also being soft is *not* desirable when someone is suffering with constipation. The primary goal is to achieve softer stools, with increased volume being a potential secondary benefit. Fermentable fibres are found in a wide range of fruit, veg, grains, nuts and pulses. So as you can see, not all fibres function the same when it comes to supporting bowel regularity, and finding the right balance for you is key.

For those dealing with constipation, it's interesting to understand that while certain high-fibre foods can enhance stool consistency and speed its journey through the gut, they typically don't have a significant impact on the muscle contractions, or peristalsis, in the large intestine. In fact, some research indicates that a diet rich in fibre may actually slow down peristalsis, potentially causing a delay in gas expulsion. The goal of including fibre is to add softness and bulk to the stool, which aids in increasing the regularity of bowel movements by reducing the time waste spends in the digestive system.

Fibre guidelines

How about we set some guidelines? Focusing on the following special characteristics of fibre can be a winning game plan if you want to beat the generic 'increase fibre and hope for the best' team.

- *Soluble and low-fermentable fibre:* Psyllium husks, along with other foods that have similar characteristics (see Fibre 1 below), are usually your best friends in resolving constipation.

- *Insoluble and non-fermentable:* Think coarse wheat bran. If you have constipation, think of these as a 'maybe' new best friend. If you're experiencing constipation with IBS however, this type of fibre is like having an old friend you don't have much in common with anymore. It's in your best interest to keep your distance, as you won't tolerate each other.

- *Fermentable fibres:* There fibres are like your support circle of friends. Each one brings something beneficial to the table, helping to increase stool size and boost the number of friendly microbes in your gut. Just like in any group, there might be the occasional odd one out – a friend who means well but can sometimes stir things up (i.e. not helping in terms of managing constipation and gut symptoms). Learning to coexist with these unique personalities is key. It's about setting the right boundaries and understanding how much interaction works best for you. Find your fibre sweet spot, just as you would find the right balance in your social circle.

When it comes to constipation relief, your goal is to find unique thresholds for all the various fibres and include enough of them to make your poo soft and formed. This will help your stool glide through your digestive system as smoothly as a sliotar sailing effortlessly over the bar, just like a spectacular score by a Limerick hurler.

It's perfectly fine to include all types of fibre in your diet if they're not mentioned in the go-to fibre foods and supplements directory that follows. However, prioritising those that are known to consistently help soften and speed up bowel movements will give you a constipation management advantage. It's also okay not to eat any of these foods if they don't agree with your gut or you don't particularly enjoy eating them.

And lastly, it's important to be aware of this crucial nugget of knowledge: boosting your fibre intake in your diet may not produce immediate or instant results. We all crave instant gratification, but it's not always achievable. Patience *is* a virtue! For some, you may start to see benefits within days, while for others, it could take weeks or even months! The important thing is not to lose hope. It will benefit your gut in some capacity in the long run.

•CHAPTER 7•
THE FIBRE FOOD DIRECTORY

Here are the foods that are more likely to address and alleviate your constipation. The pros and cons of each one are outlined. In the following chapters, we will guide you through testing them. (When amounts are in tablespoons and teaspoons, the abbreviation for 'tablespoon' is tbs and for 'teaspoon' tsp.)

Kiwi

Kiwi, that small fruit with furry skin, is making quite the buzz in the world of constipation, for easing constipation and the symptoms that come with IBS-C. There are two main commercial varieties – the green and the gold. Technically, they are referred to as 'kiwifruit', but let's just call them kiwis.

Just one kiwi is packed with almost 3g of dietary fibre, and if you have two small fruits, the recommended standard portion, that's double the fibre fix. You'll get even more fibre if you eat the skin, which is totally allowed and recommended! They're also a treasure trove of nutrients, not to mention antioxidants and phytonutrients too.

Kiwis have an amazing ability to absorb and hold on to water. If you soak a kiwi in 250ml of water overnight, it will swell to over three times its original volume. This has even been investigated with MRI machines to prove this impressive increase in water retention in both the small bowel and the colon. This water-holding capacity helps to soften the stool and can even increase how often you go – could be the easiest constipation solution you've been looking for!

Scientists are very interested in some other properties of kiwis too. One of these is the high content of something called actinidin, a type of enzyme pretty much unique to kiwis, which may help improve gut motility. Additionally, they contain raphides (tiny needle-like crystals that give kiwis their slightly prickly sensation when you bite into them), which may stimulate water secretion. Another intriguing area for research is the effect of kiwis on gut microbiota. Some early studies are showing that they might actually boost the levels of good bacteria, like Lactobacilli and Bifidobacteria, in your gut. You've got to admit, for one small fruit they are incredibly interesting! It makes you think – if kiwis are getting all this attention for their unique qualities, what other incredible characteristics might other fruits have?

What does science say?

When humans with constipation eat kiwis, a clear trend becomes evident: eating two of these green gems every day can help increase how often you have bowel movements. What's more, in about half of these studies a noticeable stool texture improvement was seen. And a really important point to note – none of these studies found that eating kiwi caused diarrhoea.

This is backed by the European Food Safety Authority Panel on Nutrition, Novel Foods and Food Allergens (NDA), which is instrumental in upholding food safety and public health standards across the European Union. They state that 'consumption of kiwifruit contributes to the maintenance of normal defecation,'* which means keeping your bowel movements regular and normal.

Even when kiwis were put to the test against other fibre champions like prunes and psyllium, they held their own. Participants eating kiwifruit saw an average rise of two bowel movements per week as well as an improvement in stool and straining and a significant decrease in bloating. Nice! More people were most satisfied with eating kiwis than any other fibre food. So it's true that two kiwis a day can keep constipation away. If you do like eating them, the key is to make a habit of enjoying those two kiwis regularly – this doesn't have to be every single day, but regularly – instead of trying them for a few days and getting discouraged if you don't see instant results.

How to enjoy kiwis in your diet

Kiwis are a fantastic fruit that you can enjoy in countless ways. Snack on them raw, blend them into smoothies, toss them into fruit salads, or dehydrate them for chewy kiwi chips. They are also perfect as a topping on your breakfast cereal or yogurt, or used in a tangy salsa. If you do eat the edible skins, just remember to wash them well beforehand!

Prunes

Prunes are like the classic, go-to natural fix for constipation, and they're deserving of their reputation. They pack a high-fibre punch, with about 4g of fibre in a serving of seven to eight prunes. Their fibre is a mix of insoluble fibre such as pectin, and soluble fibre that the gut microbes love to ferment, potentially bulking up the stool. But the real star quality may be sorbitol (already mentioned in Chapter 6), a substance known as a sugar alcohol that our bodies don't fully absorb,

---

* See 'Green kiwifruit (lat. *Actinidia deliciosa* var. Hayward) and maintenance of normal defecation: evaluation of a health claim pursuant to Article 13(5) of Regulation (EC) No 1924/2006', *EFSA Journal* 19(6), June 2021, https://doi.org/10.2903/j.efsa.2021.6641.

which helps draw water into the colon and can have a laxative effect. Prunes also contain phenolic compounds, another type of naturally occurring plant chemical, which are thought to be pretty helpful in making constipation a bit easier to deal with.

What does science say?

The scientific verdict on prunes varies, but there's certainly some promising evidence. Eating 9–10 prunes daily for three weeks resulted in softer and more spontaneous and frequent stools. Prune juice can also benefit constipation, especially by decreasing hard and lumpy stools. The good news is, no one reported having issues with loose or watery stools or terribly bad side effects with consuming prunes or prune juice.

However, it's still wise to start with a small number, say two to three per day, and gradually increase your intake to what feels like the right portion for you. Alternatively, you can opt for prune juice – begin with roughly 100ml and gradually increase it to a maximum of 200ml to help alleviate constipation. Approaching it this way will help your gut adjust to prunes and avoid any potential increase in gas, which is something people sometimes complain about. For individuals with IBS-C, prunes might pose a challenge due to their fermentability, but introducing them slowly and steadily can aid in understanding their impact.

How to enjoy prunes in your diet

To incorporate prunes into your diet, you could have them as a snack, blend them into smoothies, or mix them into salads. They can be a sweet addition to your breakfast oats or yogurt. They add a lovely depth to stews and sauces, and they can be paired with meats. They also make a great base for energy balls. Or simply drink prune juice.

Figs

Another dried fruit worth mentioning is *Ficus carica*, otherwise known as the fig. Figs, like prunes, are particularly noted for their high-fibre content, sorbitol and polyphenols. Moreover, they serve as prebiotics, altering the gut microbial community and producing SCFAs.

What does science say?

Having a daily dose of fig paste, about 10 tbs, can speed up the journey of waste through the colon in people who are constipated. It also achieves fewer hard stools and less abdominal discomfort. Interestingly, for what seems like a hell of a lot of fig paste, people did not report any specific adverse events. While you will probably find it challenging to find fig paste and actually consume that amount every day, you can find alternatives like fig 'sweets' or fig syrup in pharmacies and health food shops. It's best to use these products according to the instructions on the packet. Start with a small amount and gradually increase, assessing tolerance and effectiveness through trial and error.

It looks like figs are a good choice for those with IBS-C too, which may be counterintuitive, as they are high fermentable fibre foods, which means they may lead to increased gas and bloating for some people. In one study, about eight dried figs (90g) split between breakfast and lunch every day resulted in some lovely bowel improvements – fewer problems with constipation and abdominal discomfort. People also felt better in general. Those with IBS-C found them easy to eat, with no side effects noted. So they might be something to experiment with – again, starting slow and low and building up at your own pace.

How to enjoy figs in your diet

Figs can be easily added into one's diet. They are delightful as a fresh snack or in salads. Figs are also excellent in porridge, as a dessert topping, on gourmet pizzas, or blended into unique dips and spreads. Their sweetness also complements bitter greens and strong cheeses. When stuffed and baked, for example, with walnuts and blue cheese, they become a luxurious appetiser. Figs in baking add excellent moisture and flavour.

Mango

Mango, hailed as the 'king of fruits', could be another potential ally against constipation. It is abundant in both soluble and insoluble fibres and loaded with vitamins, minerals and polyphenols.

What does science say?

Individuals with chronic constipation who ate a large mango daily for four weeks had positive improvements in stool consistency and frequency. The mango also showed an anti-inflammatory effect, which is really interesting.

How to enjoy mango in your diet

You can enjoy mango as a fresh snack, with yogurt and other fruits. For breakfast, mangoes can enhance yogurt, cereal or porridge. They also make a great ingredient in salads – mango salsa is a fresh and delicious topping for meats or tacos. Mangoes can be mixed into rice or quinoa as an interesting side dish, and they're perfect in desserts like tarts.

Linseed/Flaxseed

Flaxseed and linseed refer to the same edible seed from the flax plant (*Linum usitatissimum*). The term linseed is more commonly used in Europe, while it's more common to hear flaxseed in America and Canada.

A tablespoon of whole linseeds – which can be either brown or golden (nutritionally the same) – contains 2.5g of fibre, making it an excellent choice for boosting one's fibre intake. The seeds are also rich in healthy fats, particularly alpha-linolenic acid (ALA) – a type of omega-3 fatty acid – and lignans, a type of phytoestrogen. Basically, you get a lot of bang for your buck!

What does science say?

When it comes to natural remedies for constipation, linseeds are another popular choice. There is some indication that consuming linseeds can markedly improve the regularity of bowel movements, reduce abdominal bloating, while also positively altering the gut's microbial composition in those who are constipated. Linseed flour, where whole linseeds are made into a fine powder using a blender, can potentially increase bowel movement frequency from twice a week to once daily (which was superior to taking lactulose solution, one of the most common laxatives on the market). People using linseed flour found it easy to use, mixing it with hot liquids such as water, milk or soy milk, or adding it to a pie recipe, which showcases its versatility and the broad range of people who may find it appealing. Variety is the spice of life.

Linseed cookies also improved constipation in those with Type 2 diabetes (remember diabetes is a disease associated with increased constipation risk). In relation to the impact of linseeds on constipation-predominant IBS, ground linseed (6–24g per day) decreased constipation and bloating after three months. In a shorter, one-month trial, 2 tbs linseeds, whole and ground, were also shown to improve IBS symptom severity.

How to enjoy linseeds in your diet

For those seeking a 'recommended dosage', add about 1 tbs of seeds, either milled or whole, brown or golden, to your diet. It's best to add them into your diet once daily, such as during breakfast, or opt for twice a day if you tolerate them well – for example, once in the morning and evening. Avoid consuming linseeds before bedtime. You can sprinkle them on breakfast cereals, yogurts, or even sandwiches, add them to soups, or use it as an ingredient in breads, muffins, and cakes.

If you observe a beneficial effect within two to three days, that's terrific! However, if there's no noticeable change, don't be discouraged

– it's still worthwhile maintaining a diet that includes seeds over the long term. Also, for anyone new to using linseeds, it's completely normal to see whole seeds in your stool, and this should not be a cause for worry!

When incorporating linseeds into your diet for constipation relief, maintaining proper hydration is non-negotiable. Aim for a total of around 2 litres of total fluid daily. To ensure that linseeds work effectively, they need proper hydration – that's 150ml extra water per tablespoon of seeds. Insufficient fluid intake while taking linseeds can, ironically, lead to constipation.

Wholegrain rye bread

Rye bread, a staple bread in many parts of Europe, not only has an interesting taste but also serves as an excellent source of dietary fibre. Just two medium slices/65g of wholegrain rye bread can pack an amazing 6.5g of fibre.

What does science say?

A large intake of rye bread daily, equating to roughly six to eight slices per day, revealed an impressive 23 per cent reduction in intestinal transit times as well as a notable increase in both the frequency and ease of bowel movements, compared with wheat bread.

How to enjoy rye bread in your diet

Rye bread is a versatile and hearty choice for meals and can be commonly found in most supermarkets these days. You have two options, normal and sourdough, and both can be wonderful. A standard portion is two slices per meal – don't feel you need eight! While we don't know if having two slices will be as effective as consuming six or eight slices of rye bread per day, eating eight slices daily isn't really a practical expectation.

How to enjoy rye bread

You can enjoy rye bread in various ways, including as toast topped with avocado and egg for breakfast. You can make a sandwich – try smoked salmon and tomatoes or Swiss cheese and sauerkraut. You can also transform it into croutons, providing a crunchy texture to salads or soups. It also pairs well with various dips, such as hummus or tzatziki.

Oat bran

Oat bran, the outer layer of the oat grain, emerges as another useful addition to a constipation friendly diet. A 1 tbs portion of raw oat bran delivers a substantial 6g of fibre. Quick oats, in comparison, contain 2.5g fibre per 30g bowl.

What does science say?

Some research has shed light on the possible positive impact of oat bran on bowel function. In one study, people who ate two oat-bran biscuits experienced increased movement frequency and consistency, along with reduced discomfort. Adding 1.5 tbs of oat bran to their daily diet also helped people reduce laxative use.

How to enjoy oat bran in your diet

For a wholesome breakfast, oat bran can be added into porridge, used in overnight oats or stirred into yogurt. It's also an excellent ingredient for homemade granola. It can be blended into smoothies, lending a fibre boost and a nutty flavour. Oat bran works well as a nutritious and texture-enhancing addition to baked goods such as muffins, bread and cookies.

Kale

Kale is a nutritious vegetable that's not just rich in flavonoids, a type of antioxidant, such as quercetin and kaempferol, but also high in insoluble dietary fibre. It is a low fermentable vegetable, which is thought to help increase the bulk of stools and thus help you go more regularly.

What does science say?

Research shows that after about four weeks of including kale in the diet, people generally saw an improvement in how often they had bowel movements. It also helps increase the beneficial bacteria in the gut and reduce the not-so-good ones. Interestingly, people who had smaller stools before eating kale seemed to benefit the most.

How to enjoy kale in your diet

You can enhance your salads with raw kale. A pro tip to improve the texture and taste raw kale is to gently massage the leaves with a good dollop of extra virgin olive oil. For those who enjoy cooked greens, sautéing kale with garlic and extra virgin olive oil makes for a wonderfully flavourful side dish. If you're in the mood for something crunchy, kale chips are a great option. Kale can also be a fantastic addition to soups and stews, where it contributes extra nutrients and a pleasant texture. Additionally, for smoothie lovers, kale is a fantastic ingredient, blending well with various fruits and adding a nutrient-rich punch.

Other potentially worthy fibre foods

In addition to the well-researched foods with proven laxative properties, there exists a range of other options rich in soluble fibre that are believed to aid digestion, although they have not been as extensively studied in human trials. Once you've integrated the more convincing 'evidence-based' foods above – that is, those with proven effects – into your diet, exploring additional high-fibre options becomes the logical next step. These foods should be introduced to your diet slowly in a bid to increase your fibre intake. Taking a step-by-step approach will allow your body to adjust accordingly. This approach not only broadens the variety in your diet but is an investment in your long-term gut health. As you reach your body's fibre tolerance, the key is to maintain this diverse array of plant-based foods in your diet. Your regular, everyday diet holds a coveted place on the podium of gut health, unlike temporary or sporadic eating habits that you might not maintain over time!

Chia seeds

Chia seeds are small, edible seeds derived from the *Salvia hispanica* plant and a member of the mint family (Lamiaceae). These tiny, oval-shaped seeds with distinct black and white specks boast an impressive fibre content, with just 1 tbs of chia seeds containing 4g fibre.

Because of their rich soluble fibre content, chia seeds have the ability to absorb 10 to 12 times their weight in water. This causes them to expand and take on a gel-like consistency. This exceptional quality not only contributes to their gel-forming ability but can also add bulk to stool.

Chia seeds are very similar in nutritional content to linseeds, but have not been formally studied in clinical trials. Instead, they have non-evidence-based TikTok research! Their resurgence in popularity followed the 'internal shower' trend, which literally took the platform by storm – the hashtag 'internalshower' has garnered over 200 million views and hopefully helped break down some poo taboo in the process! This trend promised that a blend of chia seeds, water and lemon would cure constipation. Unfortunately, some people have gone on to promote the 'internal shower' as a detox or a cleanse. It's neither of these things.

There's nothing inherently wrong with this concoction from a seed and water point of view, providing there's lots of water. Don't be tempted to swallow the seeds whole, on their own. Keep in mind also that suddenly incorporating a large amount of fibre – say 2 tbs of chia seeds – could result in abdominal discomfort, bloating and gas if your normal diet is low in fibre or you haven't had seeds in your diet before. The lemon addition is pointless and won't influence constipation (or neutralise acid!), but include it if you like the taste. Additionally, be aware that, while rare, some people may exhibit allergic reactions to chia seeds.

What does science say?

There are no trials that have looked at the impact of chia seeds on constipation. However, the nutritional qualities of chia seeds stand up in court and are recommended as part of your overall high-fibre diet.

How to enjoy chia seeds in your diet

The 'internal shower' recipe includes 2 tbs of chia seeds mixed into a large glass of water. If you're interested in trying this method, you can begin with ½ to 1 tbs of seeds and gradually increase the amount as your body becomes accustomed to it. Leaving them to soak for a while can make them easier to digest. Alternatively, you can just sprinkle 1 tbs of ground or milled chia seeds onto your meals, or you could make a creamy chia pudding with your favourite milk or use them in smoothies, cereal, yogurts or even mixed into salad dressings.

Apples and pears

Both apples and pears are fibre-rich fruits, with a medium apple providing about 2g of fibre and a medium pear providing an excellent 4g of fibre! The goodness they deliver to your gut is thanks to their natural sugars such as sorbitol and fructose, as well as pectin – a type of soluble fibre. While many people report improved bowel movements after consuming these fruits, scientific research to fully substantiate these claims is not extensive. For those unsure if they can tolerate these fruits, peeling apples and pears as well as cooking them can make them more digestible, so you could try this before cutting them out altogether.

How to enjoy apples and pears

To enjoy apples and pears, you can eat them raw, add them to salads or bake them for a warm dessert. They're also great in savoury dishes or as a sweet sauce, and even work well in soups (yes, you should try this!). Experiment by adding them into slaws or sandwiches too.

Rhubarb

Rhubarb could be a valuable addition to the diet for those suffering from constipation because of its high soluble fibre content. You know what else is interesting about rhubarb? It has this special component called sennoside that is thought to start those rhythmic contractions (peristaltic movements) that help move things along in the colon, encouraging the release of water and electrolytes in your gut too. It also has anti-inflammatory effects and can help keep your gut bugs in balance. So it's more than just an average pie ingredient.

What does science say?

Research has focused on rhubarb powder, available on prescription in Japan and highly recognised in traditional Chinese medicine. And here's a really creative idea from traditional Chinese medicine, although not available commercially yet – the invention of rhubarb navel plasters. In clinical trials, applying a rhubarb plaster right onto your belly button has shown promising results in easing constipation.

So perhaps this is a flavour of what we can expect in the future, as rhubarb has some unique plant properties. While the more down-to-earth stewed, whole rhubarb is not going to be as potent as powder form, it will still have the plant's properties in smaller quantities; so, on paper, it is a pretty good 'vegetable' to include in your diet.

How to enjoy rhubarb in your diet

While the stalks are beneficial, the leaves are toxic and should not be consumed. To incorporate rhubarb into your diet, try stewing it and adding it to porridge or yogurt, or consider using it in crumbles or tarts.

Sweet potato

A medium-sized sweet potato, especially when you eat the skin, gives you both insoluble and soluble fibre. A 100g portion of sweet potato wedges with skin on provides a very decent 5.2g of fibre. Plus, it's a medium fermentable fibre food, which means it's great food for your gut bugs. Although research is scant, with these nutritional qualities, sweet potato could help improve bowel movements and reduce constipation symptoms, and is usually very well tolerated, so it's another great addition to a high-fibre diet.

How to enjoy sweet potato in your diet

For breakfast, try them in a hash or in pancake and waffles. They can be baked, roasted, mashed with spices or made into crispy fries. They're also great in soups, stews, salads and as a grilled side. Keeping the skin on maximises their gut health benefits.

Beans, peas and lentils

When looking for affordable, fibre-rich foods that can have a substantial influence on your overall digestive well-being, beans, peas and lentils – collectively referred to as pulses – stand out as pioneers in gut health. These foods offer an abundance of dietary fibre and are incredibly versatile in various dishes. A portion – about 6 tbs of beans or lentils – provides 6g of fibre.

What does science say?

Because of their nutritional profile, pulses are a rich source of soluble fibre. They may help with increasing stool bulk, but it really is an individual thing. In one snapshot picture of eating habits, beans and pulses were associated with decreased risk of constipation. Because they are highly fermentable, they are great for your gut bugs but not so great if they trigger discomfort or pain. If introducing or increasing beans and pulses into your diet, do so very gradually and cook them thoroughly to aid digestion. Canned versions, drained and really well rinsed in cold water, tend to be easier to tolerate than dried versions, and also if you blend them – for example, in dips and smoothies. As part of your overall gut healthy diet, if you tolerate them even in small amounts, they are 100 per cent a 'yes' food.

How to enjoy pulses in your diet

Beans and pulses are so adaptable and obviously highly nutritious additions to a variety of dishes. They're excellent in soups and wonderful in creating hearty stews and curries. They are also perfect in salads, while pureed beans make for creamy dips and spreads like hummus. They can be the base for veggie burgers and patties as a flavourful, meat-free option. They enhance pasta dishes and chilli and Mexican cuisine such as tacos, burritos and wraps. For snacks, roasted chickpeas or lentil chips are crunchy options, and sprouted beans offer a unique texture in salads and sandwiches. There's nothing wrong with baked beans if they are your go-to. Indian dhals are amazing. They also help make a mean brownie!

Citrus fruit

Another trending sensation on TikTok captured the imagination with a quirky yet seemingly effective remedy for constipation, and it all started with an orange. It involves thoroughly washing the orange, cutting it into wedges, then dusting each slice with a hearty sprinkle of cinnamon and cayenne pepper. The plan? You eat the whole thing, peel and all! Now, while oranges are great, eating the peel is a stretch too far, particularly for those with sensitive digestive systems. Cinnamon adds a delightful flavour and has its own health benefits, but not for constipation, and the kick from cayenne pepper might also lead to discomfort for some. It's best to give this one a skip.

Citrus fruits such as oranges are, however, fibre powerhouses that offer a juicy, flavourful addition to one's high-fibre goals. They also contain pectin, found in the fruit's edible pulp (again, forego the peel!), which is thought to benefit bowel movement. Besides pectin, these fruits are abundant in naringenin, a flavonoid, which is a type of anti-oxidant, that has been suggested as having a laxative effect. While we don't have any human data on this topic just yet, it's safe to say that citrus fruits can be a tasty, well-tolerated high-fibre and constipation friendly addition to your diet.

How to enjoy citrus fruits in your diet

Kickstart your mornings with a fibre-rich glass of fresh orange juice, retaining the pulp for that extra fibre boost. For a nutritious snack, you can eat oranges, mandarins or clementines in their natural state or toss segments into a fruit salad or yogurt with a sprinkle of seeds for an extra fibre boost. You can also use the juice to create dressings and marinades that perfectly complement olive oil and balsamic vinegar.

Green vegetables

Kale got the limelight earlier, but what about other green vegetables such as spinach and broccoli? Despite not having concrete evidence directly connecting green veggies to better bowel function, there is a link between people eating more greens and lowering the risk of becoming constipated. It's likely because these veggies are packed with soluble fibre that helps keep things soft and your trips to the bathroom easier. So it's sensible to consider adding more greens, including kale, to your plate.

How to enjoy more greens in your diet

Spinach and broccoli fit perfectly in salads, as they do in stir-fries, roasted until crispy, steamed for a simple side, or sautéed for a quick and flavourful dish. They can also be added to soups and omelettes, and even consumed as snacks such as raw broccoli with dips. Inclusion in casseroles and baked dishes also ensures that greens can maintain a constant presence in your meals, helping to diversify your diet easily.

Summary of fibre foods

Fibre foods that have been shown to improve constipation

Food	Clinical trial to support	Recommended dose in study per day	Normal/ recommended portion per day	Constipation WITHOUT pain, bloating, gas	Constipation WITH pain, bloating, gas, and IBS-C*
Kiwi	Yes	2–3	2	Yes	Yes
Linseeds	Yes	1–2 tbs	1–2 tbs, milled	Yes	Yes
Oat bran	Yes	1 tbs	½ to 1 tbs	Yes	Yes
Kale	Yes	2 standard portions	70g	Yes	Yes
Prunes	Yes	6–8	6–8	Yes	±
Dried figs	Yes	45g	4–5	Yes	±
Mango	Yes	300g	½ medium	Yes	±
Rye bread	Yes	Up to 8 slices	2 slices	Yes	±

*People react differently to various foods, meaning some might be fine for you while others are not (hence the ± symbol in the table above). It's a good idea to try these foods yourself to see how you handle them. Start with a small amount and then gradually eat a little more over several days to find out what works for you.

Other foods that may help with constipation, but will certainly improve gut health

Food	Normal/ recommended portion	Constipation WITHOUT pain, bloating, gas	Constipation WITH pain, bloating, gas, and IBS-C*
Chia seeds	1–2 tbs, milled	Yes	Yes
Oranges, mandarin, clementine	1 medium/2 small	Yes	Yes
Rhubarb	150g	Yes	Yes
Spinach	100g	Yes	Yes
Broccoli	80g	Yes	Yes
Sweet potato	150g	Yes	Yes
Peas	80g	Yes	±
Apples	1 medium	Yes	±
Pears	1 medium	Yes	±
Brussels sprouts	80g	Yes	±
Artichoke	80g	Yes	±
Beans and lentils	120g	Yes	±

*People react differently to various foods, meaning some might be fine for you while others are not (hence the ± symbol in the table above). It's a good idea to try these foods yourself to see how you handle them. Start with a small amount and then gradually eat a little more over several days to find out what works for you – there's more information on how to increase dietary fibre in your diet in the pages that follow.

•CHAPTER 8•
FIBRE SUPPLEMENTS

Opting for a wide variety of fibre-rich foods is always a great dietary decision before reaching for supplements. That's because they are invaluable not only for their fibre content but also for the variety of nutrients they provide – vitamins and minerals, including vitamins A, C and K, potassium, magnesium and folate; and beneficial phytochemicals and antioxidants such as flavonoids, carotenoids and polyphenols. Furthermore, as we've seen, many of these foods come with their own special qualities that can lend a helping hand when it comes to easing constipation. Supplements, as their name suggests, are meant to enhance your diet, not be the sole focus. The reality is, however, that sometimes we need them.

About two-thirds of people who add a fibre supplement to their diet feel it helps their constipation (so one-third don't!). In the real world, everyone's tolerance of dietary fibres differs quite a lot, so it's important to discover what amount works for you personally. And pay heed to this extra crucial piece of information – the benefits of taking fibre supplements were seen when people took the fibre for about four weeks. It's often observed in practice that people give fibre supplements a try (or some high-fibre foods too, for that matter) for a few days, and when they see no significant changes in their bowel movements, they shrug them off as not working and call it quits. We are instant gratification creatures, after all.

So this is where it's at: fibre tends to work slowly, more like a leisurely stroll than a race. If you find yourself struggling and it appears that the fibre isn't yielding results, it's best to hang in there and continue taking it regularly, even in small amounts. However, if more fibre causes pain or you're concerned about becoming very constipated, then it's advisable to take stock of what's going on. Refer to the 'constipation wheel' illustrated in Chapter 6, page 82 to determine where you are, and seek professional support to help 'clear out'. You may just need a reset. Nonetheless, the benefits of fibre from both food and supplements are going to be better realised over the long term.

Psyllium husks

The standout fibre supplement comes in the form of psyllium husks. This soluble and gel-forming fibre is unique, making it the pièce de résistance of promoting regularity. On paper, it ticks all the boxes. It can stay intact because it doesn't ferment in the large bowel, where it keeps holding on to moisture. Say hello to bulkier, softer stools that are easier to pass.

What does science say?

Research has established the effectiveness of psyllium husks in enhancing stool frequency, weight, volume and moisture level, and in reducing the discomfort associated with passing a bowel motion. In those with IBS, psyllium husks provided significant relief, with an increase in stool weight and improved symptoms, especially in those with constipation and abdominal pain. On average, those taking psyllium husks experienced three additional bowel movements weekly, which is music to the ears of constipation sufferers. This surpasses the effect of common laxatives, which usually induce an average increase of around 2.5 bowel movements per week. In fact, psyllium husks are a type of laxative – a bulk-forming laxative – and it's widely agreed that starting with psyllium husks is the best first laxative move (see more on this in Chapter 6, page 93, and in the following paragraphs of this chapter).

Another finding is that seven types of bacteria and SCFAs showed positive changes in their numbers with psyllium husks and that these changes were particularly evident in those with constipation. This makes one think that even if you don't notice an impact with psyllium husks straight away, but you can tolerate them well, they can be a good addition to one's diet because of their microbe-changing abilities. The microbial landscape is definitely involved in constipation, even if we don't yet know the full details.

Psyllium husks: dosage and precautions

The ideal dose of 10–15g or 2–3 tsp per day has been proposed. Yes, this dose can seem like a lot to some people. The real-world view is that results can vary widely from one person to the next. You might notice a positive change with a modest 2g, while your neighbour could opt for 5g every other day, and someone else might go all-in with 10g to get the relief they're after. The key is to ease into it, gently ramping up your intake. The good news is that psyllium husks can be used for constipation and for those with IBS-C.

For example, begin with a small amount – about ½ tsp in a 250ml glass of water or juice daily. Stir well. Since the husks thicken quickly, you need to drink the mixture immediately. Consuming an additional 100–200ml of water after ingesting the husks can enhance their effectiveness in relieving constipation. You can then gradually increase the dose every three to five days, working up to 1–2 tsp per day, depending on your tolerance.

Psyllium husks are best taken in the morning, about 10 minutes before a meal (but if you forget, it's okay to take after a meal) or in between meals. To ensure compliance, it helps to consume psyllium at about the same time each day and closely monitor your body's response, adjusting as needed. Avoid taking it at night, because it can potentially cause discomfort or unwanted side effects during sleep. Additionally, it's crucial to stay well hydrated throughout the day. Expect results anywhere from one to three days after taking your first dose.

Sometimes people find that psyllium husks can lead to increased bloating and gas, and they might feel quite full. The good news is that these potential side effects can often be managed by slowly finding the dose that works best for you. It's more likely that there's an adjustment period rather than that you will continue to experience increased symptoms forever. Once your bowel gets moving, most of these symptoms may resolve. But keep in mind that since it's *your* gut we're talking about, there's a lot of individual variation. You'll need to observe and adjust the dose based on how your body responds. Your gut, your rules!

To effectively incorporate psyllium husks into your routine, it's important to find the most suitable form to help you take them consistently. If you're new to psyllium husks, know that they are available in pure form in many health food shops or online. Typically, they come powdered and in packets, featuring a light to medium brown colour and with a fine and somewhat fluffy texture. You can also buy powdered husks in flavoured sachets or mixed with other ingredients such as probiotics in pharmacies.

For those who dislike the texture as a drink, alternatives include incorporating the husks into foods like porridge, yogurt or baked items. Or you can find them in capsule or chewable versions, which bypass the need for mixing. Always refer to the package instructions to ensure you are taking them correctly. Regardless of the form of psyllium you choose, from powdered husks to capsules, always have a large glass of water ready to mix the psyllium with or drink immediately after swallowing or consuming the husks, as psyllium adores water!

If psyllium isn't helping or suitable, check out some suitable alternatives below.

Caution

Before using psyllium husks or any other supplements, consult with a healthcare provider to ensure there are no potential interactions or side effects. It's important to time the intake of husks correctly to avoid interfering with the absorption of other medications. Psyllium husks should be avoided if you have difficulty swallowing, a history of bowel obstructions, a risk of bowel impaction, or your gastrointestinal tract is narrowed. Additionally, those with kidney issues should seek advice from a medical professional before incorporating psyllium into their diet.

Wheat bran

Coarse wheat bran is the outer layer of wheat kernels, specifically the bran layer. This natural remedy owes its effectiveness to its high-insoluble, low fermentable fibre content, which adds bulk to stool and keeps it soft by retaining water to ensure regularity and comfort.

What does science say?

Coarse wheat bran has been shown to speed up bowel movements by stimulating the muscles in the intestines. Furthermore, it impacts the balance of bacteria in the gut and the substances the bacteria produce, improving the gut's bacterial composition and the by-products of the bacteria, and especially increasing the number of beneficial Bifidobacteria. Unfortunately, it's not recommended for those with IBS-C, as it can worsen diarrhoea, urgency and pain. So use with constipation but avoid with IBS-C or if you are experiencing increased gut symptoms such as bloating or gas.

How to use wheat bran

Once again, it's important to begin with a small amount, say ½ to 1 tbs, and gradually increase the quantity to give your digestive system time to adjust. As wheat bran is high in fibre, it's crucial to drink plenty of water throughout the day to help move the bran through your intestines. Aim to add to one meal a day initially, and as your body becomes accustomed to the extra fibre, you can increase or adjust as needed. Most will do well with 1 tbs per day, and a max of 2 to 3 tbs is recommended. Then give it a fair trial for at least one month, allowing enough time for the body to adjust, and see how it benefits you.

To get started, you can sprinkle it over your morning cereal or blend it into a smoothie. You can also mix it into various foods like yogurt, and it can be used in baking muffins, bread or pancakes.

When buying wheat bran, make sure you look out for 'coarse' wheat bran, as finely ground wheat bran powder works in the opposite way – it can reduce stool water content and lead to harder stools, *increasing* constipation risk! You'll probably find it easiest in a health food shop or online. It's advisable to consult with a healthcare provider before starting any supplement.

Inulin

Inulin is a fermentable soluble fibre, technically a prebiotic, which means it has a significant role in promoting the growth of beneficial Bifidobacteria while inhibiting harmful bacteria. The effect of inulin on stool consistency is thought to be linked to this fermentation process, through the production of SCFAs. This mechanism has the potential to raise the moisture levels in the digestive tract and stimulate the intestinal nervous system, which can have a positive impact on relieving constipation.

What does science say?

Positive results from inulin intake for people dealing with chronic constipation have been observed, though the way inulin does this is different from psyllium and wheat bran. Taking inulin powder may lead to improved bowel function, including more frequent stools, softer stool consistency, and a shorter time for waste to move through the intestines.

In those with IBS-C, better bowel habits and transit times were experienced when consuming inulin-enriched yogurt compared with traditional yogurt. Other concoctions with inulin in fermented milk drinks and jellies have been shown to be effective for constipation, with additional benefits in reported well-being and no negative effects. But as these products are not commercially available, it's difficult to say go out and try them!

In any case, inulin does have the backing of the European Food Safety Authority (EFSA), indicating that 12g or approximately 2 tbs per day of 'native chicory inulin' helps with the maintenance of regular bowel motions. Whether you take inulin as a supplement or not, it seems, like with a lot of things, *your* response will be *your* response.

How to take inulin

Interestingly, inulin is naturally found in various foods, including garlic, onions, leeks, asparagus, Jerusalem artichoke and dandelion greens. While not as high in inulin, bananas, whole wheat products and barley offer smaller amounts of this dietary fibre.

Chicory root stands out as one of the richest sources of inulin, and this is how you normally purchase inulin as a powdered fibre supplement. Nowadays, inulin powder is sneaking its way into all sorts of foods such as yogurt, cereal and even milk. The amount added is not always known. So, if you want to know what's really in your food, keep an eye on those labels and ingredient lists – they might give you some clues.

If you are going to experiment with inulin powder, yes, you guessed it – start with small amounts. Introducing too much inulin too quickly may lead to gut discomfort such as bloating and gas. Starting with a small amount allows your gut microbiota to gradually adapt to the added fibre. Including some inulin-rich foods in your regular diet before trying inulin powder could also improve your tolerance when introducing this supplement, as your gut microbiota may be better prepared to handle it.

When starting to take inulin supplements, some sources suggest beginning with no more than 2–3g (or ½ tsp) a day for at least one to two weeks. Slowly increase this before reaching 5–10g a day (1–2 tsp). Any side effects (for example, increased gas or bloating) should improve with continued use, especially when you titrate up slowly. But again, the response will be very individual.

Those following a low FODMAP diet (see Chapter 9, page 142) will be able to discover if these foods trigger symptoms and learn how to strike a balance between including inulin-rich foods and adhering to their dietary restrictions. Ultimately, a personalised approach is essential for managing IBS-type symptoms and still reaping the potential digestive health benefits of inulin. Plus, getting guidance from a dietitian can be incredibly valuable.

How to include more inulin-containing foods in your diet

Enjoying inulin-rich foods can be both delicious and beneficial for your digestive health. You can roast artichokes, toss dandelion greens into a vibrant salad, sauté garlic and onions to use as a flavourful base for almost all dishes, blend leeks and potatoes into a creamy soup, and grill asparagus for a quick and delicious side.

Other fibre supplements

There are a variety of other fibre supplements available, but it can be more challenging to recommend them confidently because the scientific evidence supporting their effectiveness is not as strong. However, if psyllium husks, wheat bran or inulin haven't provided the desired results, you might consider exploring some of these alternatives.

Methylcellulose

Unlike natural fibres, methylcellulose is a chemical compound and an insoluble fibre derived from cellulose. This semi-synthetic agent offers an alternative to psyllium husks. It has shown promise in helping people go to the bathroom more frequently and in enhancing the texture of stools in people with chronic constipation. It's advised to take as per packet instructions, which is usually about 5g per day.

Acacia fibre

Acacia fibre, sourced from the gum of the acacia tree, serves a dual purpose as both a fibre supplement and a prebiotic that fosters the growth of beneficial gut bacteria to aid digestion. This fibre supplement could add bulk to stool without the undesirable side effects of excessive gas and bloating. When used alongside yogurt, acacia dietary fibre helped those symptoms in IBS-C patients. Take as per packet instructions.

Partially hydrolysed guar gum (PHGG)

Partially hydrolysed guar gum (PHGG) is a natural dietary fibre that shows promise in relieving symptoms of constipation and IBS-C. Despite there not being an abundance of data available, PHGG's high-fibre content makes it a potential choice for addressing chronic constipation. Again, follow instructions on the packet regarding dosage and usage.

Fibre supplements that can help with constipation

Fibre supplement	Clinical trial to support use	Recommended dose in study per day	Normal/ recommended portion per day	Constipation WITHOUT pain, bloating, gas	Constipation WITH pain, bloating, gas, and IBS-C*
Psyllium husks	Yes	10–15g per day	5–10g (1–2 tsp)	Yes	Yes
Coarse wheat bran	Yes	1–2 tbs	1–2 tbs	Yes	No
Inulin	Yes	2–3 tbs	1–2 tbs	Yes	±
Methyl-cellulose	n/a	n/a	As per packet instructions	Yes	Yes
Acacia fibre	n/a	n/a	As per packet instructions	Yes	Yes
PHGG	n/a	n/a	As per packet instructions	Yes	Yes

*People react differently to fibre supplements, meaning some might be fine for you while others are not (hence the ± symbol in the table above). If experimenting with more supplements, try one at a time only. Start with a small amount for three days, before gradually increasing every three to five days to max recommended dose to find out what works for you.

Navigating the best supplement choices

It can certainly be worth considering some well-researched fibre supplements in the search for a constipation solution. For instance, psyllium husks have shown promise in addressing both IBS and IBS-C, while inulin may be beneficial for constipation and potentially IBS-C. Wheat bran, on the other hand, appears to be effective primarily for constipation.

Nevertheless, it's important to embrace the fundamental principle of fibre: individual responses to fibre supplements can vary significantly. Each of us is unique, and discovering the ideal solution often requires some trial and error. Personalised experimentation is the key to finding the approach that suits you best. If in doubt, a healthcare professional can help you navigate the best choices.

•CHAPTER 9•

THE FINAL WORD ON FIBRE

It's important to know that there's a difference between the findings of clinical trials and what people experience in their everyday lives. Clinical trials are carried out in a controlled and structured environment, focusing on the average or typical response of a select group of patients to a treatment. This controlled setting ensures the results are valid, but it might not capture the full spectrum of individual responses that occur in a real-world setting.

In the real world, there is so much nuance and variability among individuals – for example, in diet, lifestyle, biology, genetics, overall health and ability to comply with advice – all of which can influence how a treatment or dietary change affects a person's digestive health. It's essential to consider both clinical evidence and personal experiences when making decisions about managing constipation and finding the approach that works best for you.

Another thing you may have noticed is that in clinical trials, especially in their early stages, researchers often use higher doses of a treatment to determine its maximum tolerated dose and to observe its effects more clearly. However, these doses may not always reflect those manageable in everyday life. For example, if you were to follow a trial's advice to a tee, soon you're not going to look forward to eating eight slices of rye bread every day or 300g of fig paste, or 4 tbs of psyllium to manage constipation, because it's not sustainable or practical for everyday life! Instead, you're going to benefit from increasing the *variety* of fibre foods that have been shown to be effective, along with other foods that can work as the backroom team (covered in Chapter 10), and see their impact on you over time. There usually isn't a quick fix, but with consistent effort, you give your body the opportunity to respond.

Therefore, while clinical trials provide critical insights into the efficacy and safety of treatments under controlled conditions, understanding real-world experiences – this is YOUR response – is the most important thing. What feels right for your body and what brings you relief are what truly matter.

Navigating through this maze of dietary options can sometimes be overwhelming. Collaborating with a dietitian, especially one who specialises in gastrointestinal health, can really help. They can guide you, provide insights based on both research and practical experiences, and support you in fine-tuning your approach to managing constipation. This personalised guidance can be instrumental in helping you determine the most effective fibre sources and other remedies tailored to your unique needs. If you've increased fibre foods and you are still not happy with your stool form, you can consider a trial of fibre supplementation, as it is a low-risk, cost-effective and readily available option.

How do you know if fibre is working?

The true benefit of adding more fibre to your diet becomes clear when you notice a substantial increase in the moisture level or softness and the amount or bulk of stool you pass, and how completely you feel you've emptied your bowels. If you find that you're having more frequent bowel movements without a corresponding increase in the amount of stool or a noticeable softening of the stool, it might be a sign that your current fibre strategy isn't quite hitting the mark. Don't worry; it's just a sign that you may need to re-evaluate and make some adjustments.

For example, not going every day doesn't automatically mean you're constipated. However, frequency can't be the sole indicator of regularity. For example, someone might pass a single, hard stool daily that feels incomplete, while another person might effortlessly eliminate a large, soft stool every second day. Ironically, the daily goer is the one battling constipation, while the other is not.

For fibre to be effective, it needs to be able to soften the stool. This doesn't always affect transit. Those suffering from slow transit constipation are likely to find relief through a combination of softening the stool and accelerating intestinal movement. Achieving the right balance between these two actions can be key to resolving constipation issues. This can often be effectively managed by including fibre-rich foods in the diet (especially Fibre 1 as outlined below), some lifestyle interventions and/or introducing appropriate laxatives. Slow transit constipation can often be the most challenging constipation type to resolve, so it's recommended to approach its management under the guidance of a healthcare team. This ensures that the chosen methods are effectively integrated with any other necessary treatments and interventions, leading to the best possible outcomes.

If the root cause of constipation is related to pelvic floor muscle co-ordination, combining stool softening strategies with pelvic floor physical therapy can be a superior approach. For instance, increasing dietary fibre intake or supplementing with a tablespoon of psyllium husks, in conjunction with a dedicated pelvic health physiotherapy programme targeting obstructed defecation, can enhance bowel movement frequency.

This highlights how incorporating fibre into your diet is generally the right move for managing constipation. But for certain constipation subtypes such as slow transit or disordered defecation, a more multi-pronged intervention may be needed. Combined therapy approaches are a very cool concept for the management of conditions like constipation and IBS. In fact, this is where it's at, people. All your eggs don't need to be in the diet basket.

If fibre doesn't help, don't despair. Take it that your body is telling you something. It's time to put on your trench coat, grab your magnifying glass and start searching for more clues to unlock the secrets of constipation relief. There are various leads to explore. As said, merging different therapies and tapping into expert advice could be your ticket to relief. Keep this in mind as you navigate your options.

Fibre side effects

Fibre can be perfectly tolerated when it's consumed in the right balance and doesn't exceed what your body can comfortably handle. Some people, however, will notice some side effects, so you've got to be strategic and play around with increasing and testing fibres in a shrewd way.

For example, fibre can intensify the severity of gas and perhaps bloating and pain for some people. Insoluble fibre in particular has been linked to worsened abdominal pain and constipation, particularly if introduced abruptly and mostly for people with IBS-C, because this type of fibre is usually more fermentable.

A lot of the time these symptoms are short-lived. In fact, flatulence often diminishes as your bowel – or to be more precise, your gut microbes – adjust to the increased fibre. To ensure a smooth transition, it is advisable to – yes, you know it by now – introduce fibre-rich foods gradually into your diet, with plenty of water, allowing your gastrointestinal system to adapt effectively. It's also importance to play around with the different fibre types and amounts suitable for you, to ensure their effectiveness and reduce possible drawbacks.

Fibre supplements may also interfere with the absorption of certain medications. If you are currently taking any medications, it is advisable to consult with a healthcare professional before adding a fibre supplement to your routine.

In conclusion

Prioritising a balanced diet, high in fibre and other healthy, gut-enhancing foods, is fundamental when addressing constipation, and should always be the first line of approach before delving into other treatments. With the expanding knowledge surrounding the microbiome and gut health, our understanding has thankfully deepened. The intricate relationship between the foods we consume and the health of our gut is becoming increasingly evident. The gut microbiome plays a pivotal role in digestion and overall gut functionality. Consuming a diverse range of nutrient-rich plant-based foods not only provides essential fibre but also nourishes these beneficial microbes, supporting optimal gut health. As such, the emphasis on a balanced diet isn't merely a traditional or anecdotal recommendation; it's firmly rooted in emerging scientific insights into gut health. The summary of foods for managing constipation provided here should offer optimism and opportunities for individuals searching for natural approaches to alleviate their condition.

Summary of fibre considerations

1. **Effectiveness of fibre types:** Not all fibres are equally effective. For instance, certain insoluble fibres may not offer significant relief.

2. **Side effects:** Though generally safe, fibre can cause some discomfort such as bloating, gas and abdominal pain. You have to discover the right fibre balance for you.

3. **Quality of evidence:** Although fibre is often recommended for chronic constipation, the quality of supporting evidence is not always top-notch. This is likely related to the design of the trials rather than any shortcomings of fibre itself. It can be very effective in the real world.

4. **Personalised recommendations:** A general advice to 'eat more fibre' can be too broad and confusing to implement for many. Working off the fibre lists that follow will help you figure out which specific foods work best for you and will help you determine if increasing fibre will be effective. If it doesn't give you satisfactory relief, don't worry; there are plenty of other strategies to explore, as discussed in the upcoming chapters.

5. **Matching fibre to constipation types:** Fibre will likely work well for the majority. But it may not work as well for those with slower digestion or problems related to stool evacuation. This is certainly not to say that increased fibre won't help slower transit and evacuation disorders – softening the stool is always advised. But addressing these types of constipation usually needs more of a team effort that involves physical therapy (pelvic floor physio), medical consultation (doctor or gastroenterologist) and dietary guidance (dietitian) to enhance your chances of achieving effective relief.

How do I get started with increasing fibre?

The following two comprehensive tables try to do the hard work for you so you can know the right fibre choices and find the right balance. This first table, Fibre 1, focuses on soluble fibres with low to medium fermentability. These foods should have the most positive impact on your bowel regularity. and are a great place to start when trying to increase fibre and manage constipation, especially if you have IBS-C or any associated constipation symptoms like pain, bloating or gas. In this book, this list of foods is referred to as 'Fibre 1'.

Fibre 1

Fruit	Vegetables	Grains	Pulses	Nuts & seeds
• **Kiwi**	• **Kale**	• **Oat bran**	• Tofu	• **Linseeds/ flaxseeds**
• *Rhubarb*	• *Sweet potato*	• *Oats*	• Tempeh	• *Chia seeds*
• *Orange*	• Carrot	• Rice bran	• Quorn	• Sunflower seeds
• *Grapefruit*	• Spinach	• Quinoa		• Peanuts
• Ripe banana	• Aubergine	• Wholegrain rice		• Walnuts
• Passion fruit	• Turnip			
• Raspberry	• Broccoli			
• Strawberry	• Green bean			
	• Beetroot			
	• Potato with skin			

Foods in bold text are those with convincing clinical evidence. Aim to include these foods regularly in your diet. *Foods in italics are similar in terms of their fibre properties, and can likely help.*

The list also includes other foods beyond those highlighted in bold and italics, which also have beautiful fibre and plant-based properties, with possible softening effects, offering you a way to include a broad selection of these foods in your diet. Know that you're not restricted to just the bold and italics for life, although these can be prioritised. Incorporating a diverse range of foods rich in fibre is recommended, as this variety is likely to enhance your overall gut health long term.

Now, let's move on to another selection of fibre-rich foods, which we'll call 'Fibre 2'. These are all wonderful foods, as they are considered prebiotics, or food for your gut microbes. And as your microbes may be involved in helping improve transit through the bowel, you want these in your diet. However, the foods in Fibre 2 are distinct from those in Fibre 1 in relation to how easily they ferment. Fibre 2 foods are high fermentable fibres, so if you find that bloating and gas are troublesome companions to your constipation, it's wise to introduce these foods gradually into your diet. Use the guidance below to help increase these in your diet. For those who are severely constipated or in pain, it's advisable to hold off adding these foods until you become more regular.

Fibre 2

Fruit	Vegetables	Grains	Pulses	Nuts & seeds
• **Prunes and prune juice**	• *Peas*	• **Rye bread**	• *Lentils*	• Almonds
• **Figs**	• Brussels sprouts	• Barley	• *Chickpeas*	• Pistachios
• **Mango**	• Avocado	• Wholewheat bread	• *Black beans*	• Cashews
• *Pear*	• Asparagus	• Wholewheat pasta	• *Kidney beans*	
• *Apple*	• Sauerkraut		• *Butter beans*	
• Blackberry	• Artichokes		• *Baked beans*	

The foods listed in bold are the ones backed by clinical evidence, so you know they're reliable additions to your diet. Aim to include these foods regularly in your diet, as tolerated. *Foods in italics can help manage constipation – include these too.*

Again, don't feel like you have to stick only to foods that are in bold or in italics, even though they can be your go-tos. Including as many as you want and can tolerate is the best approach for your gut health in the long term. Finding the perfect balance of fibre that works for you is the goal.

Increasing fibre – perfection!

When you're considering increasing your fibre intake, consider the lesson from the tale of the tortoise and the hare: taking it 'slow and steady' leads to victory. If you zoom ahead like the hare and pile on the fibre too quickly, your gut might protest – you might need to lie down with all the increased gas and bloating you experience. Instead, be the tortoise – increase your fibre gradually over weeks or months. This gentle approach gives your digestive system the time it needs to adjust, so you are crossing the finish line with a happy, regular gut.

Increasing fibre

Go low ... → And slow ... → Drink plenty of water!

When you're increasing your fibre intake, start with a small portion of the food. Choose the foods that you like and would find it easy to consume regularly in your diet. If you're experiencing many gut symptoms or feeling anxious, consider starting with half of the usual portion size. In this case, it's advisable to initially choose only one food from Fibre 1. However, if you're dealing with constipation *without* additional gut symptoms like bloating or gas, you have the flexibility to select any food from either Fibre 1 or Fibre 2. The aim is to increase by one fibre food every five to seven days.

As you progress, continue to gradually introduce new foods into your diet on a weekly basis, focusing on those that are more likely to soften your stools. The ultimate goal is to incorporate two to three fibre-rich foods into each meal and include fibre with snacks as well. If you don't manage the full whack, that's okay. Keep adjusting until you find what works for you and also helps soften your stools. Sometimes, small changes can go a long way. Continue this process until you consistently experience effortless and complete bowel movements.

Example of how to increase fibre for constipation

Week 1	Week 2	Week 3	Week 4
Linseeds: ½ tbs × 3 days, increasing to 1–2 tbs/day	**Kiwis:** × 1–2/day	**Prunes:** 2 prunes, increasing to 4–8 per day	**Psyllium husks:** ½ tsp increasing to 1–2 tsp per day

If you find that a new food consistently causes increased gas or bloating, it's a good idea to temporarily remove it from your diet. You can try reintroducing it later when your bowel movements are more regular. Remember, fibre is most effective when it's combined with adequate water intake. You can find more details about this in Chapter 11. As always, it's best to consult with a healthcare provider before making any major dietary changes, to ensure they align with your personal health needs.

Case study (fibre balance)

Meet Olivia, a sociable 34-year-old who attended the Gut Health Clinic because she had been dealing with constipation, gas and bothersome bloating for some time. She needed a solution.

Exploring Olivia's diet: Olivia had always been conscious of her diet and had made such a great effort to include plenty of fibre-containing foods in her diet. However, despite her best efforts, this did not lead to less constipation or fewer symptoms. When we dug a bit deeper into her diet, we noticed something interesting. While Olivia was eating a wide variety of plant-based foods, there was an imbalance between the types of fibre she was consuming. She had more of the insoluble and fermentable kind (e.g. pasta, wheat cereal, pulses) and less of the soluble kind (especially fruit, as she felt fruits were too high in sugar!). It was also noticeable that her total fluid intake was low.

The plan: The approach with Olivia was all about balance and making gentle adjustments to her diet. It was important not to advise her to give up her favourite foods or go on a restrictive diet. Instead, it was recommended to *add more* low fermentable soluble fibre sources (you know them now as Fibre 1) to her daily routine to address the suspected root causes of her discomfort.

But there was a crucial piece of advice: as Olivia increased her fibre intake, she needed to make sure she was drinking enough water, especially with linseeds, as these guys are like little sponges that need water to work their magic.

The outcome: The changes Olivia made might sound simple, but they had a profound impact on her bowel. She was thrilled to discover that she didn't have to say goodbye to her established diet – or worse – follow a restrictive diet. By introducing soluble fibre, with a focus on two kiwis per day, 1 tbs of ground linseeds in the morning, and more fruit overall, as well as staying hydrated, Olivia experienced the desired improvements. The most significant change for Olivia was the relief she felt. She started having regular morning bowel movements, and her bloating became a thing of the past. She was back in control.

Olivia's story shows us that even small dietary adjustments can make a big difference in how our bowel works and in how we feel. It reminds us of the power of personalised dietary guidance and how it can transform our overall well-being.

(Side note: Understand that insoluble and more fermentable fibre foods are really enjoyed by your gut microbes. Instead of ever thinking about eliminating these fibre foods completely, first aim to change the balance of fibre in your diet. Incorporate more soluble fibre-rich foods first (Fibre 1). If this does not work, then gradually reduce insoluble, more fermentable fibre foods (e.g. Fibre 2).)

I'm afraid to increase fibre – what should I do?

Understandably, the thought of increasing fibre in your diet can be intimidating for some people, especially if they've concerns or fears about how their body will react. You know, some people will have already tried upping their fibre intake, just like the usual advice suggests. They might have gone for a generous helping of brown pasta and ended up with stomach cramps or gas. Others might vividly recall the fallout after eating a meal loaded with fibre, for example a stew, curry, soup or smoothie that left them bent over in pain. Others may have tucked into a veggie burrito on a whim, having avoided beans for the past year. Never again! Past encounters like these can leave a lasting impression, instilling a sense of total reluctance and sometimes avoidance when it comes to boosting fibre intake.

These past experiences of digestive discomfort or even embarrassing moments can be internalised and make us fearful of attempting to increase our fibre intake. And it's entirely reasonable to have these concerns. But here's the important part: when it comes to boosting your fibre, it's all about proceeding at your own pace, with care … and a plan.

You deserve to feel comfortable and in control throughout this journey. Remember, it's not a race, but a thoughtful and gradual process. The key to increasing fibre is to do so with caution and empathy, prioritising your comfort and maintaining a sense of control throughout the journey. Going from zero to a hundred overnight, especially when dealing with any food anxiety, fear or gut symptoms, isn't the way to go. It's like handling delicate glassware – you need to treat the situation with kid gloves.

If you find yourself in this situation, feeling fearful, anxious or stressed about increasing your fibre intake, the best approach is to take it very, very slowly. Deliberately and mindfully increasing fibre in your diet at a gradual pace can lead to better outcomes. Begin this process with a thoughtful self-assessment of your current dietary habits – look back at your food and symptoms diary. Take some time to consider which foods you would like to add to your diet. Selecting foods that suit your taste preferences is crucial to making this transition enjoyable and sustainable.

My list of food challenges

Challenge	Food	Reason for excluding food in the past
1		
2		
3		
4		
5		
6		
7		
8		
9		
10		

Then start to challenge with a selected food, using a very small portion. This can be as little as one-fifth to one-third of a normal serving, like just 1 tbs of mashed sweet potato or 1 tbs of chickpeas, as it will allow your digestive system to adapt gradually. It also builds your confidence as you observe how your body responds, and it will minimise any severe reactions. As the weeks progress, slowly increase the portion size towards a normal portion for you. For example, increase by 1 tbs at a time, all the while attentively observing how your body responds. This will allow you to find how much of that food you tolerate. This can take days, weeks or even months, but you are in the driving seat, so there's no need to rush it. Staying patient and persisting with smaller amounts for as long as needed is perfectly acceptable. Create your own style. Once you know your tolerance level of a food, keep including that food in your diet. Then start a new challenge.

If you ever feel bad after trying a new food, stop the challenge right away. The amount you managed the day before you felt a reaction is probably what your body can handle for now. But if the symptoms are just a bit uncomfortable, try to stick with it – your gut might just be getting used to this food again. Or, you can keep having the same smaller portion a few more times before bumping it up. Before you jump into another food challenge, give yourself a little break, like a three-day respite, until you're feeling better. And when you're ready, start challenging with another food. Your body might surprise you with what it can get used to over time.

Maintaining as varied a diet as possible while challenging is recommended throughout your fibre-increasing journey, and keeping a food journal to track your progress and any discomfort can provide valuable insights. It's also going to be helpful to seek guidance from a registered dietitian, as personalised support can be immensely beneficial. Remember, you are in control, and this journey is about nurturing your well-being at your own pace.

Example of a food challenge, e.g. bread

Time	Portion	Symptoms
1st challenge	¼ slice	No symptoms
2nd challenge	½ slice	No symptoms
3rd challenge	¾ slice	Mild bloating
4th challenge	1 slice	Mild bloating
5th challenge	1½ slices	Worsening bloating and wind.*
6th challenge	Stop challenge	
7th challenge		

* As you can see, this person will be able to tolerate one slice of bread without major gut upset. Having more than that triggered symptoms. Over time, the amount of bread tolerated can increase. But for now this person can enjoy one slice and reduce any anxiety related to eating this amount of bread.

Now it's your turn. You can use the following template example.

Time	Portion	Symptoms
1st challenge		
2nd challenge		
3rd challenge		
4th challenge		
5th challenge		
6th challenge		
7th challenge		

My tolerated fibre foods

Foods I can eat freely	Foods I can have in smaller amounts	Foods I don't tolerate very well at this time (I'll try to eat this food again in 3–6 months' time)

Case study (fibre fear)

Meet Evelyn, who came to the Gut Health Clinic with debilitating symptoms and increased food anxiety. She was experiencing severe pain, bloating and flatulence, and she was never able to fully empty her bowels. Although she didn't think she was constipated because she was passing small amounts of stool every day, they were type 1 on the Bristol Stool Chart (which, as you know now, fits the criteria for being constipated!).

Evelyn had been cutting out various foods from her diet over the previous couple of years in an attempt to manage her symptoms. Her diet had become quite limited in variety and fibre – she avoided most grains, fruits and pulses. She had also cut out dairy, which led to low dietary calcium intake. She was drinking plenty of water – over 3 litres per day, in the quest for better digestion. She was committed to regular exercise, hitting the gym five days a week and walking 10,000 steps a day. Her weight was stable, but anxiety and stress easily got the better of her.

The plan: The plan for Evelyn was to make gradual changes. We agreed to slowly increase her intake of soluble fibre using Fibre 1. We discussed which foods she'd like to reintroduce into her diet and created a plan. She also introduced deep belly breathing before meals (10 long, slow breaths with a longer exhale) to help her relax and help manage food anxiety (refer to Chapter 13, page 199 for detailed instructions on how to perform deep belly breathing). To address her low calcium levels, she started to include lactose-free options. We also suggested reducing her water intake, as excessive water intake doesn't provide any extra constipation benefits (see Chapter 11 for more explanation on this).

Outcome no. 1: When Evelyn returned for her follow-up appointment four weeks later, there were some very positive changes. She had successfully introduced five soluble fibre foods into her diet: kiwi, raspberries, linseeds, quinoa and kale. Her stools were softer, and her bloating, gas and incompleteness had improved, although they were still annoyingly present. Evelyn asked about following the low FODMAP diet, a restrictive diet for IBS (see page 142).

It was felt that jumping into the low FODMAP diet right then might have been a bit too much for Evelyn, even though it could really help with her symptoms. See, her diet was already pretty low in FODMAPs, and she was dealing with quite a few dietary restrictions. Plus, it seemed like anxiety was playing a big part in what was going on with her, which means the low FODMAP diet was not the best fit for her at that time. Instead, we stuck to our plan of slowly upping her fibre intake, and this time we added in psyllium husks. Evelyn was super open to trying this out, especially now that she had a good grip on what a few small but tailored changes can achieve.

Outcome no. 2: The real breakthrough came when we slowly introduced psyllium husks. It made a profound difference, and Evelyn's bowel movements became consistently complete. The joy of a complete bowel motion was exquisite! Her symptoms had also mostly reduced, with some fluctuation from time to time. Evelyn connected her symptoms to stress and anxiety. She agreed to explore gut-directed hypnotherapy to further address these factors (see more on this in Chapter 13, page 195).

Evelyn's journey was a testament to the power of gradual changes and finding the right solutions tailored to her needs. With continued support and strategies to manage stress, she was well on her way to a constipation-free life and overall well-being.

IBS with constipation (IBS-C)

Navigating the world of IBS can be like walking through a maze with multiple turns and dead ends. However, the good news is that treatment of IBS has made great strides over the past number of years, and there are clearer paths towards accurate diagnosis (check out the diagnostic criteria in Chapter 3, pages 26–27 for a quick recap) and approaches to tackle this tricky condition.

Here's a ray of hope for those with IBS with constipation (IBS-C): the food you eat is a powerful ally in your journey to wellness. Here are some ground rules for IBS-C.

1. Establish regular mealtimes and take your time eating; rushing can upset your digestive system.

2. Avoid long gaps between meals to keep your digestive system in sync.

3. Hydrate with at least eight glasses of water or other non-caffeinated beverages throughout the day.

4. Moderate your intake of carbonated drinks and alcohol to minimise bloating and irritation.

5. Limit your intake of tea and coffee to a maximum of three cups per day to prevent potential digestive discomfort.

6. Choose fewer processed foods and ready-to-eat meals, and avoid reheated foods, as they can make symptoms worse.

7. When it comes to fruits, moderation is key; aim for no more than three servings per day to maintain balance. Also spread your fruit out throughout the day.

8. Prioritise increasing your intake of soluble fibre, which can be particularly beneficial for your bowel movements and overall gut health – Fibre 1 is a good place to start.

These dietary approaches and often simple adjustments can be very effective in the overall management of IBS-C, but are unfortunately overlooked in favour of restrictive diets. They are, however, what people with IBS-C should work on *before* they start cutting foods from their diet! Fibres can be key players in all of this when you know which ones to choose. While soluble fibre is typically beneficial, insoluble fibre may not be as beneficial and could worsen symptoms – for some individuals. The goal is to identify the type of fibre that your body responds to positively. Fibre 1 should help manage IBS-C without making symptoms worse, with most people being able to enjoy some if not all foods from Fibre 2 as well.

As outlined already in this book, the key is to tailor your diet to your personal needs. It's a process of experimentation to find what agrees with your body. What helps one person may not necessarily help another. Approach your IBS-C dietary management as a journey of exploration. Keep an open mind and be willing to adjust your food choices. This approach isn't just about managing symptoms – it's about enhancing your overall well-being and navigating the complexities of IBS with confidence. With IBS-C, the 'trial and error' game *is* the process. What's a hit for one might be a miss for another.

FODMAP restricted diet and fibre in the management of IBS-C

The above 'ground rules' can be highly beneficial for at least half of people who suffer with IBS. If these recommendations don't yield results, it might be appropriate to follow a restrictive plan known as the low FODMAP diet. FODMAP is an acronym for some specific types of carbohydrates – Fermentable Oligosaccharides, Disaccharides, Monosaccharides and Polyols. In susceptible individuals, these particular carbohydrates can give one's digestive system a tough time, leading to not-so-fun things like bloating, gas, stomach aches and altered bowel habits. This low FODMAP diet works for between 50 and 80 per cent of those who try it.

The FODMAP diet is supported by trusted groups like the British Society of Gastroenterology and the American College of Gastroenterology. So, what's the deal with this diet? Well, it's all about playing detective with your food. You start by taking a break from foods that are high in FODMAPs (sometimes all high FODMAP foods, sometimes a subset of high FODMAP foods), usually for two to four weeks. Then, if you respond (that is, your symptoms reduce), you bring them back into your diet one at a time to test your reactions to each one. This way, you can identify which high FODMAP foods might provoke symptoms and in what amounts, and which ones do not.

For most people, it's usually just a few specific high FODMAP foods that cause issues. The ultimate goal is to pinpoint your trigger foods while still enjoying a varied and nourishing diet. If you can tolerate a food in small amounts, rather than avoiding it completely, it's best to include it in your diet in those small amounts. The idea is that by including small amounts of foods you tolerate, over time, this may improve your tolerance to those foods, which can be comforting to know.

For those wrestling with constipation issues, it's worth noting that a low FODMAP diet, often suggested for IBS sufferers, can be a double-edged sword. While it can help reduce symptoms like painful stomach cramps and bloating, it can also lead to reduced fibre intake.

This decrease in fibre might affect the amount of softness and bulk in your stool, or how your intestines draw in water and how your gut bacteria process certain foods, which could increase the risk of constipation. While this is certainly not observed in everyone with IBS-C, it's crucial for those considering this diet (especially for those already facing constipation) to work closely with a knowledgeable dietitian to strike the right balance.

Indeed, working closely with a dedicated dietitian plays a huge role in the success of the low FODMAP approach. Your dietitian will provide personalised guidance to tailor the diet to your specific needs, making it easier to navigate this somewhat complex dietary journey. It's worth knowing that, alongside fibre, following a low FODMAP diet could potentially lead to deficiencies in important nutrients such as calcium, B vitamins and iron. However, your dietitian will ensure that these essential nutrients are maintained in your diet. They will also guide you to avoid excessive restrictions, such as eliminating entire food groups.

Additionally, dietitians are instrumental in addressing eating behaviours, including disordered eating and eating disorders, which are relatively common among individuals with IBS. Their expertise goes beyond just the diet itself and encompasses your overall health and well-being.

The low FODMAP diet has been observed to reduce the presence of some species of bacteria, such as Bifidobacterium, which are beneficial for gut health. While experts don't fully understand the implications of this, when you follow the low FODMAP diet correctly – that is, firstly restricting these foods temporarily (for no more than six weeks) and then gradually reintroducing them to find your personal threshold level – the levels of these bacteria tend to stabilise once again. This means you will minimise any negative impact on your gut microbiota when following the low FODMAP diet correctly.

Multiple studies have consistently demonstrated that people experience improved long-term symptom management and reduced need for additional interventions when they receive guidance and support from a dietitian while following a FODMAP diet. Those who attempt it independently often face challenges in implementation and express a desire for dietitian guidance. The aim is to find a middle ground that helps ease your symptoms while ensuring you get all the nutrition your body requires – all the time still enjoying your meals.

Conclusion IBS-C

In an ideal world, we would have a simple fix for IBS-C, but unfortunately, it's not that straightforward. It can't be because of the nature of the condition. According to current knowledge, the initial step for both constipation and IBS-C is to work towards softer stools by incorporating more soluble fibre into your diet and staying well hydrated – focus on getting that stool out! If this approach doesn't yield the desired results, the next step may involve a personalised strategy, such as a customised low FODMAP diet. If this resonates with you, and you haven't already consulted with a dietitian as part of your healthcare team, now is an excellent time to consider doing so.

Case study IBS-C

Mark is a hardworking individual who came to the Gut Health Clinic seeking relief from severe pain, bloating, reflux and bowel issues, with mostly type 1 and type 2 bowel movements on the Bristol Stool Chart. Mark's daily life was really busy, with his full-time job, caring for his elderly parents and his home life, leaving little time for himself. Despite trying a gluten- and dairy-free diet, he didn't experience much improvement, and his feeling was that maybe they made things worse.

During the assessment, we discovered that Mark's diet was high in FODMAPs, even though he was still excluding two major culprits – wheat and dairy. Stress also played a potentially significant role in contributing to his symptoms.

Plan 1: To address this, we agreed a plan for a modified low FODMAP diet, focusing on removing the most commonly consumed high FODMAP foods to make it manageable given Mark's busy schedule. We agreed on suitable food swaps and provided him with a meal plan, recipes and snack options. Mark decided to bring his lunch to work, as it was more convenient than eating out, especially as it's challenging to navigate a FODMAP diet out and about.

He also started practising mindfulness for just 10 minutes a day to help manage stress, using a popular app. He found the plan realistic and was eager to implement it.

The outcome: Upon his return, Mark had experienced satisfactory relief from his symptoms. He suspected that garlic, apples and maybe even sugar-free chewing gum were his main triggers. He also became more in tune with the tension in his body, which he knew was due to his busy lifestyle, and acknowledged the importance of mindfulness.

Plan 2: The next step in Mark's journey was to proceed with the re-introduction phase of the low FODMAP diet, where he would gradually reintroduce the six previously omitted high FODMAP foods over approximately six weeks to better understand his tolerance to each one. Mark understood that even if he tolerated these foods only in small amounts, it was better to keep them in his diet rather than exclude them altogether, as the situation is dynamic, meaning tolerance can change over time.

Additionally, he committed to continuing his mindfulness practice, recognising its significance for long-term management.

In the end, Mark was delighted with the plan's effectiveness and felt more in control of his digestive health. It was a journey of understanding, acceptance, and finding the right balance for his unique needs.

• CHAPTER 10 •

BEYOND FIBRE – OTHER FOODS THAT MAY HELP ... OR HINDER

Other foods that may help

Healthy fats

Are you familiar with the notion that healthy fats can help 'lubricate the stool'? If so, it's important to clarify that this idea is somewhat exaggerated and may have been inspired by the effects of certain laxatives like paraffin oil. While these laxatives do provide lubrication, they are derived from petroleum and differ significantly from the healthy fats found in foods. Nevertheless, despite a lack of research in this area, there are some arrows pointing towards the fact that healthy oils could be effective for constipation, possibly by increasing the frequency of bowel movements and softening the stool.

To make sense of the potential benefits of healthy fats for constipation, it's a great idea to incorporate a variety of healthy fats into your diet – for example, eating oily fish twice a week, along with nuts, seeds, avocado and extra virgin olive oil. If these healthy fats were to have a stimulatory effect on the bowel, then it might be sensible to include them at breakfast, as that's the time when bowel contractions are typically strongest. For example, you could add some nuts or nut butter to your cereal or enjoy avocado and an egg fried with extra virgin olive oil on toast. Why not experiment and see if this works for you? It just might, and your gut bugs will certainly thank you.

Fermented foods

Fermented dairy products such as yogurt, kefir and pickled vegetables have been a staple in human diets for centuries. They are created by friendly microbes that work their magic on foods to transform and reinvent the ingredients into microbe-rich delights. They have traditionally been used to aid in food preservation. However, fermentation also unlocks more nutrients and removes toxins in food, boosting the food's nutritional power.

When it comes to constipation, scientists are still unravelling what fermented foods might contribute to our gut. Human trials are needed to figure out which fermented foods and how much can make a difference. They may possibly help constipation, but no one is confident yet to say which ones and how much a person might use to get an effect.

There is a hint of evidence suggesting that yogurt may help with constipation and that sauerkraut may lessen the severity of symptoms in people with IBS. Kefir is possibly the most promising fermented food. It is a probiotic-rich fermented milk drink, and several small trials have looked at its impact on constipation. It led to the need for fewer laxatives and improved stool consistency in those who were in hospital and also suffering with constipation. Drinking 500ml of kefir per day (a large volume!) led to a notable increase in the number of bowel motions, improved bowel satisfaction score, and a reduction in gut transit time in both normal transit and slow transit constipated folk.

Two months of consuming kefir led to a notable reduction in constipation, abdominal pain and bloating, and diminished the frequency of gas. But because of study design flaws, we're unsure if this was a placebo effect – was the reduction in constipation after drinking kefir because the people drinking it believed it worked rather than that the kefir itself worked?

There is also a kefir elephant in the room: every batch of kefir can have a unique mix of microbes. If you prepare your own kefir using your unique grains, the microbial composition will be distinct from that of John's down the street, who uses a different set of starter grains, leading to variations in the kefir's characteristics. This variation in microbial content from one batch to another complicates our understanding of kefir's health effects, because you're not evaluating an identical product each time.

How to enjoy kefir and yogurt in your diet

That said, kefir can be incredibly versatile in the kitchen, and yogurt and kefir are probably the best fermented foods when you have one eye on constipation. Both kefir and yogurt can be blended into a smoothie or poured over your cereal in place of milk for a tangy twist. You can also use them to make a creamy salad dressing or a dip for veggies by mixing in herbs and spices. Or you can simply enjoy them on their own. If trying kefir for the first time, it's advisable to take a small amount and gradually increase intake, especially if you have gut symptoms along with constipation or IBS-C.

If you want to try kefir, there's the commercial option, produced under controlled conditions, offering consistency but possibly less microbial diversity. Or, if you're feeling a bit adventurous, why not make your own kefir? It's pretty simple – just get some kefir grains and mix them with milk. Voila! You'll have your very own homemade batch, which usually has more varied microbes than commercially prepared versions.

Yogurt may be beneficial, particularly those labelled as 'live' or 'bio' – words that indicate the presence of beneficial microbes. For example, cows' milk yogurt, strained yogurts like Greek and Nordic yogurt, as well as non-dairy yogurts with 'live' cultures on the label, can all provide gut-health benefits.

Foods that may hinder

Foods that may contribute to constipation: truth vs myth

Two foods are frequently assumed to be connected to increased constipation, namely bananas and cheese. Let's debunk!

Bananas

Bananas are a popular and excellent fruit, known for their nutritional value and convenience. The impact of bananas on constipation is influenced by their ripeness. Unripe, green bananas contain high levels of what's known as resistant starch, which can be harder to digest and could perhaps contribute to constipation in some individuals. As bananas ripen, this starch transforms into simpler sugars and the fibre content becomes more favourable, which could help improve bowel regularity and stool consistency. Therefore, while unripe bananas might be constipating for some, ripe bananas are generally beneficial in managing constipation as a result of their soluble fibre content. One small to medium size ripe banana is therefore okay.

Cheese

The belief that dairy products – especially cheese – cause constipation is widespread, yet there's no solid scientific proof to back this up. Of interest, elderly residents in a retirement home who ate more cheese did not become more constipated. In fact, there was no noticeable change in bowel activity, transit time or gut symptoms. The absence of dietary fibre in cheese does not necessarily mean it contributes to slowing down digestion. Instead, cheese is valued in a balanced diet for its contribution of energy, protein and vital micronutrients such as calcium.

Moreover, cheese is increasingly recognised for its benefits to gut health. Specifically, it contributes to microbial richness. In one study, cheddar cheese – especially porter-soaked cheese, provolone and Swiss cheese (cheese lovers' cephalic phase of digestion should kick in about now) – topped the cheese microbial diversity table. Interestingly, the cheese rind boasts the most significant microbial richness, so you can eat both the cheese and its rind. Be sure to avoid the wax or cloth on some cheeses, however.

If you enjoy cheese, you can still include it in your diet, balancing the consumption of cheese and other dairy products with a higher intake of whole plant foods to continue to promote regularity without compromising the intake of crucial nutrients.

While it's wrong to dampen the spirits of dedicated cheese enthusiasts, it's a good idea to be somewhat informed about cheese portion sizes. While individual responses can vary, there's no need to completely forego the cheeseboards. Standard serving sizes for cheeses are:

- Hard and semi-soft cheese is about 25g, roughly the size of a matchbox.

- Soft cheese is about 50g.

- Cottage cheese or ricotta is about 75g.

Constipation-friendly cheeseboard

2–3 strong, preferably smelly cheeses; fresh berries or dried fruits; an assortment of nuts; wholegrain crackers; and a dollop of plum or quince jam.

High-fat diets

Generally, high-fat diets are linked with increased constipation. But as some evidence suggests, healthy fats may help to reduce constipation. So it seems that just like fibre, not all fats are created equal! Saturated fats, like those in butter and fatty meats, are the ones thought to slow things down. They might even upset the balance of good bacteria in our gut by reducing microbial diversity and promoting bacteria linked to inflammation and gut diseases.

Saturated fat is found in foods like a full Irish breakfast, burgers and fries, deli meats, fried chicken and steak with chips, or potatoes with lashings of butter. However, most people don't usually consume large helpings of these types of foods daily. What's more commonly seen is where you consume a large portion of meat in a meal, which then limits how much space you have for fibre-rich foods such as vegetables, whole grains and legumes.

The ketogenic diet, generally rich in fat and low in fibre, has often been associated with constipation. However, the opposite has also been reported: a high-fat diet sped up transit, leading to diarrhoea. Plus, not everyone who eats a high-fat diet is constipated (or has diarrhoea), so there's more to the story than singling out fat.

A shift in dietary balance to more animal products and less fibre could possibly be the link that leads to an increase in constipation. But is it the high fat or the lack of fibre that's the issue? We don't know exactly! So to avoid any potential constipating effects, it's advisable to reduce overall saturated fat intake, increase the healthy fats, balance your diet with plenty of fibre-rich foods, and maintain adequate hydration.

Clues as to what could be happening so far are only available from animal studies. But it appears that with a diet high in junk food there was a worrying decrease in the number of cells responsible for releasing serotonin (the enterochromaffin cells), and also in the actual levels of serotonin. In addition, even the genes involved in creating and moving serotonin changed. And with less serotonin around, things can slow down a lot, leading to slower digestion and more frequent bouts of constipation.

Other insights include how fat can change the rhythmic contractions in the bowel. After a high-fat meal, there were some reverse rhythmic contractions, potentially slowing down the journey of food through the colon, which doesn't happen with carb-heavy meals. In another experiment, when a fatty solution was introduced into the gut it took nearly three times longer for things to pass through a certain section. This also made the gut stretch out and move less than usual. However, it's important to note that these processes are complex and can vary from person to person.

Fat intake and IBS

People with IBS often have a more sensitive gut, known as hypersensitivity. This means that their gut responds unusually to normal things that typically don't cause discomfort. For example, the digestive system's response to high-fat foods, which would not typically provoke symptoms in a healthy person, may cause discomfort or exacerbate symptoms in someone with IBS, indicating a heightened sensitivity to fats. So it's generally advised to limit fatty, greasy, creamy and processed food if you have IBS.

Refined grains

Refined or 'white' grains are more quickly digested compared with whole grains. Examples include foods like white breads, rice and pasta, as well as white flour used in packaged snacks. These grains are stripped of many of the wholegrain nutrients during processing, which cuts down on their nutritional goodness substantially.

In one estimate, almost all of the fibre content and over half of the B vitamins are lost when refining wheat to produce a fine flour ideal for breads and pastries. Even if certain nutrients are reintroduced through fortification, it's impossible to restore the full spectrum of beneficial components found in whole grains, including phytochemicals – the amazing plant chemicals lurking in the outer layers of the grain. So more whole grains and fewer refined grains are the sensible choice. Use your fibre tables to help gauge what wholegrain foods suit you and your constipation most.

Ultra-processed foods

Recently, there has been growing interest in the impact of ultra-processed foods (UPFs) on gut health. While not all processed foods are detrimental, many UPFs are devoid of amazing fibre, your trusted companion when dealing with constipation. Adding to the concern are the high levels of saturated fats, trans fats (another unhealthy fat) and artificial sweeteners (think sugar-free products) in highly processed foods. Another thing is that they're also usually high in salt, which has been highlighted as a constipation foe too. It's speculated, but not proved in humans, that UPFs both alter the gut bacterial balance and directly irritate the intestinal lining. So really, there's nothing positive to say here!

But for those challenged with constipation, reducing the intake of processed foods and embracing whole, fibre-rich foods is probably a proactive step towards achieving regular bowel movements and maintaining gut health. Opting for browsing the fruit and vegetable aisle and buying whole grains such as rice, quinoa, oats and breads, as well as a variety of nuts, seeds and pulses in their natural form, will reduce the presence of UPF ingredients in your shopping trolley.

Overall diet/habitual eating

Researchers have looked at how well people's overall diets reduce the risk of constipation. It has been shown that for people consuming more of certain foods – specifically total fruits, whole fruits, total vegetables, greens and beans, whole grains, total protein foods, seafood and plant proteins – there was a reduced risk of constipation.

While some studies have delved into the link between specific foods and constipation, one can't deny that in daily life we eat meals composed of a mix of foods and therefore nutrients, rather than isolating specific ones. Therefore, in addition to incorporating fibre-rich foods that aid in alleviating constipation, adopting a healthy eating regimen will likely enhance your overall constipation-relief strategy.

Conclusion

Making all the relevant suggested dietary changes can be a great way to say farewell to constipation for many people. But – and there's always a nutritional *but* – they might not provide complete relief for all. So first, remember to take your time with changing your diet. Slow and steady wins the race! Second, sometimes the positive effects may take a while to manifest, so patience is key. In any case, these dietary adjustments are not only good for constipation but are also beneficial for your long-term health. So when you make then, you've nothing to lose and everything to gain by keeping them in your diet. If you find this challenging or continue to experience stubborn gut symptoms, a dietitian is there to help you figure out what's going on.

Next up is the chapter about fluids, which will help you nail your dietary plan. Then get ready for more insights, as the upcoming chapters could offer the additional winning solutions you've been looking for to cut down your time in the bathroom. It's time to broaden the horizons, explore all angles and uncover a multitude of other ways to help manage constipation.

•CHAPTER 11•

FLUID AND CONSTIPATION

Hydration

Water is the primary component of our body, making up about 60 per cent of our total weight, and it plays a vital role in almost every aspect of our bodily functions. This includes regulating our body temperature, facilitating chemical reactions, maintaining blood volume, and aiding in transporting nutrients and removing waste. If our body doesn't get enough water, our life can be detrimentally affected – we basically shut down within three days. We don't have the option to go fluid-less.

Our bodies are quite amazing at regulating water levels, typically fluctuating by less than 2 per cent each day. If you lose more than 1–2 per cent of your body weight in water, you're entering dehydration territory. This level of dehydration is often associated with symptoms such as increased thirst, dry mouth and darker urine. More than 2 per cent can lead to more severe symptoms and health complications if not addressed promptly.

Curious to know how to assess your hydration levels? Just look at the colour of your urine. If it's clear or pale yellow, you're on the right track with your hydration. On the other hand, if it appears dark yellow, that's the sign to increase your water intake. And if your urine appears brown, it's a significant indicator of dehydration: boost your water consumption immediately.

Are you drinking enough fluid?*

Adult women should aim for 2 litres per day.

Adult men should aim for 2.5 litres per day.

*Fluid includes water and other beverages that hydrate the body.

How best to hydrate

Water is obviously the best choice. It's important to maintain a balance in your beverage choices by incorporating plain water and other hydrating fluids to ensure adequate hydration. But if plain water doesn't excite your taste buds, and you're on the lookout for other thirst-quenching alternatives, rest assured; hydration isn't limited to just H_2O. Caffeinated drinks also contribute to total fluid intake! Herbal teas, fruit-infused water, coconut water, vegetable juices and milk (including dairy and plant-based varieties) are all excellent caffeine-free options for staying hydrated. People also get water from the food they eat, and it is reckoned that this can contribute approximately 20 per cent of our overall water intake. Vegetables and fruit are especially high in water – cucumber and lettuce are approximately 96 per cent water, carrots and broccoli 88 per cent. Yogurt, interestingly, is 80 per cent water and boiled eggs are 75 per cent water. Some biscuits contain just 3 per cent water!

Let's rewind to the mention of coffee (and tea) being hydrating. There are numerous myths about coffee, and one persistent belief is that it causes dehydration. However, regular coffee drinkers who had four 200ml servings of coffee with 4mg/kg caffeine (280mg caffeine for a 70kg man) showed no notable difference in their hydration status, which confirms that consuming coffee in moderate amounts doesn't lead to dehydration.

However, when caffeine is consumed in high amounts, more than 500mg or approximately six coffees per day, caffeine can act as a diuretic, meaning it may increase urine production. For the average person, therefore, enjoying a few cups of coffee a day can be part of a healthy hydration strategy without concerns about dehydrating effects. But don't use this as a justification to rely on caffeinated drinks for most of your fluid requirements either! Pay attention to your own body's hydration status and ensure a balanced intake of various fluids throughout the day.

It's interesting that while we all feel thirsty occasionally, in everyday life thirst isn't always the primary driver for our fluid intake. More often we consume liquids as part of our regular meals and snacks. Additionally, many of us enjoy drinks like tea and coffee, not just for hydration, but for the delightful pick-me-up and social opportunities they create.

Our body signals thirst in two main ways. When we lose water and the concentration of salts in our cells increases, our brain detects this and makes us feel thirsty. Additionally, certain brain sensors react to changes in our body's water levels, becoming more active when salt levels are high. Surprisingly, even the taste of water can trigger these sensors, indicating our body's proactive response to hydration needs.

The water balancing act

The amount of fluid we drink impacts our body's hydration, but the speed at which we rehydrate depends on various factors, especially how quickly these fluids reach the parts of our intestines where absorption takes place. On average, it can take about 20 to 30 minutes for water to pass through the stomach and enter the small intestine. However, smaller volumes of water may pass through more quickly, while larger volumes, or more concentrated drinks, or water consumed with a meal, may take longer.

Imagine someone drinks about 1.5 litres of hydrating fluids and gets around 400ml from their food each day. Our digestive system surpasses that amount as it actively releases a roughly estimated eight litres daily – approximately four times the combined intake of fluids and water from food. This liquid includes gastric juices, bile, pancreatic fluids and intestinal secretions – all essential for digestion.

Most of the liquid gets absorbed while still in the small intestine, which can handle up to 15 litres every day! The colon, our brilliant defender against constipation, absorbs about five litres daily. These amounts do vary from person to person, and things like what you eat and how well you're hydrated can make a difference. The intricate balance of fluid intake, absorption rates and bodily processes ensures that our body remains properly hydrated and capable of carrying out essential functions, like the desired soft and smooth bowel movements.

What does science say?

It might come as a surprise that the connection between water consumption and constipation isn't fully understood. What's equally unexpected is that individuals with chronic constipation often have a similar fluid intake to those without constipation! So, as with most things to do with constipation, it's not always a straightforward connection.

Digging deeper, however, it appears that those who drink the fewest fluids are more susceptible to constipation. An interesting study revealed that men who reduced their daily fluid intake from 2,500ml to just 500ml began to experience constipation. Apart from staying hydrated, the link between a high-fibre diet and increased fluid in managing chronic constipation is definitely one to pay attention to. Individuals who included 25g of fibre in their diet and raised their daily water intake to 1.5 to 2 litres experienced notable improvements in their bowel regularity. This suggests that when fibre interacts with water, it may lead to more frequent bowel movements. The question arises, however, is it the fibre alone working its magic, or is it the combination of fibre and water?

Not all research agrees, however. Two studies didn't find a significant link between increased water intake and better bowel movements, whether people drank extra water or included more water with a fibre supplement. So how water intake affects constipation treatment has yielded mixed results. The key takeaway is that maintaining adequate hydration is crucial, and combining water with fibre appears important too. However, going overboard with hydration, or overhydrating, does not appear to provide additional benefits. For example, increasing water intake from 2 litres to 3 litres is not going to enhance bowel activity.

Also, an excessive amount of fluid might lead to a sensation of bloating. Rather, sipping water steadily throughout the day can enhance the body's absorption of fluids and help reduce the bloated feeling associated with consuming large quantities of liquid at once.

How much to drink?

Sometimes our body's thirst signals aren't the best at telling us when we need to hydrate. Things like being active, hot weather or certain health conditions can increase our need for fluids, but we might not always feel thirsty right away. So, it's a good idea to get into the habit of sipping water throughout the day, even if you're not feeling super thirsty. Maybe start with a glass of water when you wake up, have one with each meal, and keep a water bottle handy during the day. Find what works for you.

Aiming for around six to eight glasses a day, or roughly 1.5 to 2 litres of non-caffeinated drinks, is usually a good bet (and checking the colour of your urine can be a handy guide to see if you're on track). And oh, when you're bumping up the fibre in your diet, remember to hit that fluid goal – it will really help!

'Bad water drinker' tips

Create habit	**Morning drink**	**Download app**	**Alternate with caffeine**	**Flavour**
Get in the habit of keeping a water bottle with you throughout the day.	Bring a large glass of water with you to bed and drink first thing upon waking.	Download a 'drink water' app, e.g. Daily Water, Water Reminder, Plant Nanny.	For each cup of tea or coffee, alternate with a glass or water or cup of herbal tea.	Flavour water with e.g. strawberries, basil and lemon, cucumber and mint leaves, orange and thinly sliced ginger, pineapple chunks and sliced lime.

Mineral water

Epsom salts, which are magnesium sulphate, have a long history as a remedy for constipation. In fact, the medicinal properties of magnesium sulphate were recognised and patented as far back as 1818. Magnesium has been shown to have a laxative effect when ingested in high doses, as it draws water from the intestinal walls and softens the stool, helping to relieve constipation (see more in Chapter 16).

Recent research has focused on the constipation-reducing effects of mineral waters rich in magnesium sulphate. Three European brands – Hépar, Ensinger Schiller Quelle and Donat Mg – have been studied for their influence on functional constipation, with people drinking from 500ml to 2 litres per day. While some of the research so far suggests that mineral water rich in magnesium can help with constipation, the overall results are not entirely convincing. This may change with future trials, however.

Just a heads-up, if you're thinking of giving mineral waters a try, especially those with high magnesium levels, you might find it a bit tricky to find them. They're not on your regular supermarket shelves. Plus, imagine if you needed up to 2 litres a day – that's a lot of water to have to import!

Coffee

Views on coffee's role in health have dramatically shifted over recent years. Where it was once seen as a perceived health risk, it is now viewed as a potential protector. This globally cherished beverage boasts a rich array of bioactive compounds including polyphenols and diterpenes, and it has been associated with numerous health benefits. Early lab tests, animal studies and surveys suggest that coffee may offer several benefits to the digestive system. These benefits include its role as an antioxidant, its capacity to reduce inflammation and its positive impact on gut motility.

In addition, because of its thousands of plant compounds, coffee has been shown to have a positive influence on our gut microbes. Both caffeinated and decaf coffees, especially when roasted, can impact the levels of certain bacteria in our gut, notably increasing the numbers of beneficial bacteria such as Bifidobacterium. The effects appear greater the more coffee is consumed.

This is perhaps due to its soluble fibre content – yes, coffee contains fibre – but the amount is relatively minimal compared with high-fibre foods like fruits, vegetables, whole grains and legumes. It could also be related to a number of polyphenols, which are types of antioxidants. Nevertheless, the full landscape of coffee's influence on the gut remains mostly uncharted territory.

Coffee and digestive movement

Here's a brief overview of what we know so far, and keep in mind that the effects can vary considerably from person to person.

Positive effects

Almost 30 per cent of healthy people have an increased urge to have a bowel motion shortly after coffee (black, unsweetened) consumption. This urge can come as quickly as four minutes after and remain visibly higher for at least half an hour after sipping their brew. This suggests that the effect is produced by triggering the gastrocolic reflex (see Chapter 2, page 18) in the stomach and small bowel, because coffee can't actually reach the large bowel in four minutes. The effect was higher in females. Interestingly, hot water had no effect on the urge to move bowels.

In another study, again in non-constipated people, participants were given three different drinks – a cup of hot, black, caffeinated Colombian coffee, decaffeinated coffee and water – and a 1,000-calorie meal (a very large meal!). Caffeinated coffee was found to greatly enhance movement in the colon, leading to more contractions. These contractions were similar to having a meal, 23 per cent more effective than decaf coffee, and 60 per cent more effective than water. Consuming caffeinated coffee appears to stimulate the colon roughly to the same extent as eating a meal, and it does so significantly more than either water or decaffeinated coffee.

So it looks like coffee's link to chronic constipation is inverse, meaning it doesn't cause constipation but could actually help alleviate it for some people. The exact coffee components causing these effects haven't been pinpointed. Although caffeine is probably contributing to these effects, it doesn't seem to be the full story. There's a suggestion that coffee might stimulate the release of certain gut hormones such as cholecystokinin and gastrin, which are involved in the gastrocolic reflex, which then would increase the urge to poo.

Negative effects

However, coffee isn't all about good news for everyone. It can lower the pressure in your lower oesophagus and ramp up stomach acid production. This might lead to heartburn for some. And while caffeine can kickstart colon activity, it's not always the best choice for those dealing with diarrhoea or incontinence – it's too much of a good thing in those cases. Also, for folks with IBS, coffee can be a bit of a mixed bag. Sure, it might help with constipation, but it can also worsen symptoms such as bloating and cramps for some. Plus, caffeine has a knack for amping up stress and anxiety, which isn't great for IBS symptoms. And let's not forget about sleep – caffeine can really mess with it, both in terms of quality and how easily you nod off, especially if you're sipping it too close to bedtime. If you're finding this to be true, try to wrap up your coffee time by early afternoon, say around 2 o'clock, or even noon for the extra sensitive among us.

Drinking coffee for constipation

If you experience a coffee-induced bowel movement boost, it can be a delightful morning treat. As you begin your day and get moving, your colon also starts to wake up. Consuming coffee in the morning, alongside all the other recommended morning rituals you will find in this book, can help improve the chances of a regular and glorious morning bowel movement. The effects of tea are unknown, so it's best to test this out for yourself if you prefer tea over coffee. In any case, a hot, caffeinated drink in the morning will contribute to your overall fluid intake and help keep you hydrated – another constipation win.

Juice

Constipation fibre guidelines recommend the intake of whole fruits, including those high in sorbitol. Juice that contains sorbitol – particularly varieties like prune, apple and pear – has also been known to offer relief when feeling 'stuck' (see more on this in the fibre directory in Chapter 7). While there's often concern about the sugar content in fruit juices, when consumed in moderation and as part of a balanced diet these natural sugars can sometimes be beneficial for those struggling with constipation. As always, it's advisable to choose 100 per cent natural juices without added sugars or preservatives.

How to include juice in your diet for constipation

- Keep the serving size small, with a maximum of 150ml per day.
- If you're constipated, try prune, apple or pear juice.
- If you're constipated and experiencing pain, bloating or gas, opt for orange or grape juice.
- Juice is better used as a short-term constipation solution than a regular 'must-have' addition to your diet.

Alcohol

Alcohol has a wide range of effects on the gut, and unfortunately none of them is particularly positive. Sometimes, going overboard with alcohol can worsen constipation, as it can slow down intestinal movement and disrupt its normal functioning. Higher alcohol content in drinks might increase the likelihood of this. For others, alcohol can have the opposite effect, speeding up digestive transit and seeming to alleviate constipation. Some people with constipation find that alcohol helps 'clear them out', likely because of this speeding up motility effect. However, using alcohol as a solution for managing constipation is not something that can be recommended!

Excessive alcohol consumption can lead to dehydration, another factor that we now know contributes to constipation. Moreover, too much alcohol can disrupt the healthy balance of gut bacteria, potentially leading to bacterial overgrowth and increased intestinal permeability, aka leaky gut.

While an occasional drink may not immediately trigger digestive problems, regular and heavy alcohol use can contribute to ongoing issues, including constipation. Have you noticed that alcohol exacerbates your constipation? If so, reducing your intake or avoiding alcohol might be beneficial.

If you do decide to enjoy a drink, it's a good idea to keep in mind the recommended national guidelines for alcohol consumption:

Women: less than 11 standard drinks per week.

Men: less than 17 standard drinks per week.

A standard drink typically refers to:

   half a pint of beer

   100ml of wine

   one pub measure (approximately 35.5ml) of spirits.

•CHAPTER 12•
EATING BEHAVIOUR

Meal pattern

Your bowels are incredibly smart and can thrive on routine. The key message when it comes to constipation is that skipping meals, especially breakfast, is not advisable. Here's why.

Eating initiates the gastrocolic reflex, the process by which consuming food signals to the stomach to inform the lower intestine to clear the way for new food and helps set off mass movements in the intestines (remember we covered this in more detail in Chapter 2). Governed by the enteric nervous system (your 'second brain', in your gut), these movements often lead to the urge to defecate after eating. They are particularly active and stronger in the mornings, likely due to the body's circadian rhythms – more on this below. Therefore, skipping meals, particularly breakfast, means missing out on an opportunity to sync with your body's built-in signals and natural rhythms.

However, proving this is difficult. There have been some reports where some individuals practising intermittent fasting reported becoming constipated. This may be because missing a meal disrupts the regular stimulation of the digestive system. However, not everyone experiences this effect. It's possible that those who are already prone to constipation might be more likely to experience an increase in not being able 'to go' when fasting. During Ramadan, when for those who observe it there's a big change in eating habits due to fasting, there seems to be a risk of increased constipation too. Those who fasted were about twice as likely to experience constipation compared with those who didn't fast. What's more, people who fasted for two weeks or longer were three times more likely to have severe constipation symptoms than those who fasted for a shorter period. This kind of hints at a connection between fasting, including not eating in the morning, and an increased chance of becoming constipated.

Although not directly associated with constipation, there is another important gut process worth mentioning in relation to your eating behaviour and gut movement: the migrating motor complex (MMC). The MCC primarily functions in the small intestine to help clear undigested food, bacteria and other substances out between meals. The cycles of the MMC typically occur every 90 to 120 minutes and continue during fasting states – including the periods between meals and throughout the night. When you eat, this process is interrupted to make way for the newly ingested food. The digestive system then shifts focus to breaking down and absorbing nutrients from the recent meal, temporarily halting the MMC activity.

If the MMC doesn't have the opportunity to complete its cycles because of constant eating, it might lead to digestive issues. If you are a grazer and/or a nighttime snacker, this cleaning wave activity can be disrupted, potentially making overall digestive movement slower. On the other hand, prolonged fasting periods between meals allow the MMC to function more effectively. A more structured eating pattern, say the norm of eating meals every three to four hours, will allow for adequate fasting periods between meals, which should optimise the MMC, helping it initiate more cleansing waves and clear the small intestine.

However, this is not a strict rule. Some, particularly those with IBS-C, may prefer a schedule of smaller, more frequent meals. And that's OK. You will need to figure out your own individual preferences and responses. Balancing meal frequency with your needs is key, and consulting with a healthcare provider or registered dietitian can provide personalised guidance for improved digestive health.

The sensible approach to help the overall management of constipation is to stick to three regular meals each day, which can help support the proper functioning of these natural digestive processes – the gastro-colic reflex, mass movements and the MMC. Establishing a daily routine of three meals – breakfast, lunch and dinner – at more or less the same time each day is likely to be more effective for helping constipation than skipping meals and grazing throughout the day. For those prone to constipation, it seems especially important to work with these natural processes, not against them. It's therefore worth reflecting on your meal patterns, such as meal timing, frequency, snacking habits and nighttime eating. Consider whether changes in your eating behaviour could assist in managing constipation more effectively.

Three golden rules of eating behaviour

Eat regularly: 3 meals/day.
Avoid grazing

Meal spacing: Eat every 3–4 hours (but have a snack if hungry).

Overnight fast: Avoid eating late at night. Aim for a >12 hr overnight fast, from last meal until breakfast, e.g. dinner at 7 pm, breakfast at 8 am.

Circadian rhythm

Have you heard about our body's internal clock, also known as the circadian rhythm? It's getting a lot of airtime in the science world these days because it appears super important in managing almost everything about our health and well-being. Imagine it like an internal 24-hour timer that keeps our body functions and behaviours on track, in response to the natural light–dark cycle. There's this master controller in our brain that makes sure all our organs are in sync with this rhythm.

This circadian rhythm has a significant impact on regulating a range of gut functions, including the production of gastric enzymes and fluids, the absorption of nutrients in the small intestine and the movements of the stomach and intestines. It also influences sleep patterns, hormone release, eating habits, body temperature and many other important bodily functions.

There's a growing recognition of the importance of maintaining a regular eating schedule to support our natural circadian rhythm, leading to better mental and physical health outcomes, with an emphasis on a lifestyle more attuned to our body's natural rhythms. In fact, 'chrononutrition' is a relatively new field of study that combines principles from chronobiology – the science of biological rhythms – with those from nutrition. It focuses on the timing of food intake and how it aligns with the body's internal clocks, particularly the circadian rhythm. The core idea is that it's not only *what* you eat but *when* you eat that can significantly impact your health.

Your colon, as mentioned before, also follows a circadian or 24-hour pattern. It is characterised by a state of rest during the night and a sharp increase in activity upon waking, with ongoing activity throughout the day. This rhythmic pattern, governed by internal biological clocks, prepares the body for expected events like meals. When this circadian rhythm in the bowel is disrupted, it could be another chink in the system that increases the risk of constipation.

Our circadian rhythm or body's internal clock can get a bit mixed up. You see, when we eat plays a big part in keeping our daily life on track, both in terms of our body's clock and our social routines. Take shift workers, for instance. Their eating schedules and habits often change – they might eat more high-fat and carb-heavy meals, and often these meals are grabbed quickly, eaten cold during short breaks. This can lead to more snacking, more often on pre-packed stuff and more sugary or caffeinated drinks. Besides struggling with sleep, a big thing shift workers often face is tummy trouble – anywhere from 20 to 75 per cent experience this, and it's constipation or IBS that's most prevalent. Makes you think about how important our eating routines are, right?

Travellers are another cohort susceptible to a disrupted circadian rhythm. Crossing multiple time zones can lead to what is known as jet lag – a classic symptom of disturbed circadian rhythm – but also 'traveller's constipation', as abrupt changes to mealtimes (and sleep!) can affect the digestive process. As mentioned, the altered eating schedule during fasting can also influence gut function and potentially lead to constipation-related challenges. So, as you can see, the timing of meals and the natural functioning of the gut are closely intertwined.

As you can now gather, the absence of regular meals could potentially impact the gastrocolic reflex, MMC and large bowel contractions, all of which are influenced by the body's circadian rhythm. One approach that is believed to improve our internal clock's function and potentially alleviate constipation is maintaining consistent mealtimes. Shift workers can support their circadian rhythm and bowel health, despite irregular schedules, by adopting several strategies. It's crucial to eat at consistent times each day, aligning 'breakfast', 'lunch' and 'dinner' with the start, middle and end of the shift, respectively. It's also recommended to avoid large, heavy meals, caffeine or alcohol before bedtime.

Other factors that can help support one's circadian rhythm include regular sleep – including going to bed and waking up at the same time every day, even at weekends – to reinforce your body's sleep-wake cycle (see Chapter 13, page 205, for more on this). Incorporating relaxation and stress management techniques such as deep breathing, meditation or gentle yoga can be a big help in winding down before bedtime.

Additionally, exposure to natural light, particularly in the mornings, is beneficial, as sunlight plays a significant role in regulating circadian rhythms. It's also important to manage your exposure to artificial light in the evenings. Bright screens and artificial lighting can disrupt your body's perception of day and night, so consider using blue light filters on your devices. Engaging in regular physical activity, ideally in daylight, can further synchronise one's circadian rhythms, although vigorous exercise close to bedtime could be overly stimulating.

When people are in dim light instead of bright light during the day, their bodies don't absorb as much carbohydrate from their evening meal, even though their internal body clock times seem the same. This suggests that being in dim light during the daytime can slow down the digestion of an evening meal, causing some of the food components not to be absorbed properly.

Moral of the story: Spend time in natural daylight. Sunlight helps regulate your circadian rhythm, which is connected to optimal digestion.

Chewing food

Have you ever been in such a rush that food doesn't even touch the sides? Do you ever eat on the fly, shoving down a sandwich between meetings? Have you mastered typing with one hand on the keyboard while the other hand feeds the mouth, all while staring at the screen? Or skipped the lunch queue and resorted to liquid lunches or energy bars

– the kind of food that barely needs chewing? If this sounds familiar, don't worry – it's just a part of being human in our fast-paced world. Eating slowly and chewing your food thoroughly is often not taken seriously when it comes to digestion, but this could be important.

Chewing is the first step in the complex process of digestion (see Chapter 2, page 14). Its role as a hard grafter, doing the heavy lifting before the stomach and intestines get all the glory, is normally very underappreciated. In general, most of us are too accustomed to rushing through our meals, when we should be trying to chew our food thoroughly, reducing it to a pulp-like consistency, before swallowing. Faster chewing and fewer chews per mouthful are associated with a larger meal intake. It's quite a stretch to say that overeating is the reason you are constipated, but rapid eating and inadequate chewing during overindulgence can hinder proper digestion. Moreover, high-calorie, low-fibre food choices are more common with overeating, neither of which are desirable when the bowel is acting up.

Properly chewing your food is a wise move so that you prepare your stomach to digest food effectively. Eating too quickly or not chewing enough means that larger food particles end up in your stomach and intestines. Neither your stomach nor your intestines are equipped or designed to handle the job meant for your teeth and saliva. As a result, swallowing food or drinks without sufficient chewing demands more digestive effort and poorer nutrient absorption.

Even though there isn't a ton of research on it yet, there was a study with older people who chewed gum. Turns out, chewing gum helped them with salivation and passing gas, and even made bowel movements a bit easier compared with those who didn't chew gum. So there's a thought – that maybe chewing can give our gastric motility a little boost. In some situations, people who chew gum after bowel surgery help get their gut moving again by reducing gas and making it easier to go to the bathroom. However, do note that it's not the gum that's interesting but the act of chewing – it's possible that it tricks your body into thinking you're eating, which could potentially stimulate bowel movements. To be completely honest, the effect is likely minor, but it's interesting all the same.

For individuals with IBS, it's important to be cautious with gum, especially sugar-free chewing gum. Although its mild laxative effect from artificial sweeteners may seem advantageous, these sweeteners can actually worsen gut symptoms like bloating or gas in some people. While chewing gum is not harmful, it's worth noting that it doesn't provide any substantial nutritional value to the body.

Studies involving non-human subjects have shown that diets consisting of powdered food, which requires no chewing, result in constipation-type symptoms, including slower colonic motility. When subjects switched back to regular diets that necessitated chewing, there was an improvement in the constipation-like symptoms and a reduction in colon inflammation.

Eating slowly and chewing more also helps prevent overeating. It also activates the parasympathetic nervous system (more on this in Chapter 13, page 185), which supports digestive processes, including managing blood flow in the gastrointestinal tract. However, individual differences such as health status and stress levels mean the exact digestive benefits of slow eating can vary from person to person.

So chewing is most likely beneficial from a holistic standpoint and is intertwined with optimal digestion and stress responses. While some experts suggest chewing each bite 30 times, it's not helpful to be counting to 30 each time we take a mouthful of food. Instead, try to approach it mindfully. The key is to chew your food thoroughly until it reaches a soft, pulp-like consistency (think porridge) before swallowing. This simple yet effective habit not only enhances digestion but also allows you to savour your meals thoroughly and derive maximum satisfaction from your eating experience.

Mindful eating

Mindful eating involves engaging all of our senses, extending beyond just the sense of taste. As conscious beings, every sense we possess, including smelling, seeing and touching food, significantly contributes to our overall eating experience. Mindful eating involves consuming food with a sense of non-judgemental awareness, redirecting one's focus towards the act of eating and the connection between the mind and body.

It also involves identifying emotions connected to food, such as anxiety stemming from past digestive discomfort. It has been proven that mindful eating is effective in addressing unhelpful eating habits such as ignoring cues of hunger and fullness, and in easing digestive problems related to stress. While it may not have a direct effect on constipation, mindful eating can positively influence eating behaviours, which could, in turn, provide some relief for constipation issues. Additionally, thorough and mindful chewing has been shown to reduce stress eating, curb cravings and enhance fullness feelings.

To get a sense of mindful eating at home, you could engage in simple exercises that heighten your sensory awareness. For instance, you might slowly chew a slice of crisp apple, focusing on the crunch and the burst of sweetness with each bite. Or you could take a moment to enjoy the aroma and temperature of a freshly brewed cup of coffee or maybe a herbal tea, noticing the subtle flavours as you sip it. These activities encourage you to be fully present and attentive to your eating or drinking experience, fostering a deeper appreciation for the food and drink, and its sensory qualities, thereby promoting mindful eating.

To enhance the mindful eating experience, it can be beneficial to create an environment that supports relaxation. This can be done by setting the table and making sure the dining area is free from clutter. Additionally, introducing a calming element, like a candle or music, can enhance the atmosphere and further encourage mindful eating.

Tips for being more mindful when eating:

- When it's time to eat, why not put down your phone and switch off the TV? Try to keep distractions to a minimum. Also, eating while you're on the go or driving isn't the best idea. It keeps you in that 'always alert' mode of your nervous system, which isn't desired for digestion. So, taking a little time to relax and focus on your meal can be a gut-positive move.

- Before your first bite, take a moment to appreciate the presentation and aroma of your meal. This sensory experience triggers emotional pleasure and stimulates the release of saliva and digestive juices, preparing your body for digestion.

- Why not take a moment to express some gratitude and do some deep belly breathing (check out Chapter 13, page 199 for this)? This little ritual is really great to nudge your body into a relaxed state, perfect for optimising digestion. Chewing your food to a pulp-like texture before swallowing is a good rule of thumb.

Mindful eating emerges as a versatile and effective strategy to enhance digestive wellness, complementing other health-improving habits. At its core, mindful eating plays a significant role in digestion through stress reduction. By incorporating mindful eating into your everyday routine, you can develop a positive relationship with food, reduce the likelihood of both overeating and undereating, and ultimately give yourself a better chance of optimising your overall digestive function. And who knows, it may aid and certainly won't hinder your battle with constipation.

Hunger fullness scale

To properly understand your food choices and eating patterns, it's important to recognise the crucial role of hunger and satiety signals in beginning digestion. A useful method is to use a hunger scale prior to starting a meal, assisting in understanding your body's signals. This strategy can prevent both overeating and undereating, enabling you to become more conscious of what motivates your eating. Is it physical hunger or emotional factors, for instance?

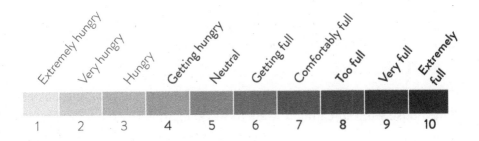

Visualise a hunger scale ranging from 1 to 10, where 1 is extreme hunger and 10 is feeling extremely full. Ideally, you should avoid both extremes. When you're hungry, approximately at a level 3, is believed to be the best time to start eating. Engage in mindful eating – savour each bite and keep an eye on how full you're feeling. Hitting around a 7 on the scale, where you're full but not stuffed, can help prevent overeating. But hey, we're all human, right? So it's totally okay if you're not always starting your meal at a 3 or finishing at a 7. Remember, this isn't a strict rule, but more like a friendly guide to help you tune into your body's own signals.

An interesting point is that skipping meals can lead to extreme hunger, possibly reaching a 1 or 2 on the scale, which often results in eating too quickly and not chewing properly, which in turn may be counterproductive for digestion. Taking the time for self-reflection (in your head or in a journal) before meals can deepen your understanding of the internal and external influences on your eating habits. To gain a clearer insight into your relationship with hunger and fullness, consider asking yourself these sample self-inquiry questions.

- How do I feel emotionally before, during and after eating (e.g. stressed, overwhelmed, bored, hungry, lightheaded, tired)?

- Am I aware of the production of saliva in my mouth before I take the first bite?

- Are my feelings primarily linked to physical sensations, emotional states or a combination of both?

Case study: Constipation morning routine

Details

Joan is a serial five-minutes-to-get-ready kind of gal, dashing out of the house without eating to walk to work, logging on to her computer, only coming up for air and downing a cappuccino at eleven. Her main complaint when attending the Gut Health Clinic was constipation with severe bloating.

Assessment

Joan's diet and lifestyle were thoroughly evaluated. Despite her diet being rich in beautiful plant-based foods and healthy fats (her lunch and snacks were excellent!), and despite being well hydrated, walking to work and enjoying regular hikes at weekends – and feeling stress-free for the most part – one particular aspect of her routine stood out: she never had breakfast. This pattern began when she started her professional career, as early morning commutes left her with little time to sit down for breakfast. She was also more of a night owl than a morning lover, so getting up earlier did not appeal, and anyway, she never really felt hungry first thing in the morning.

The plan

Joan agreed to start incorporating breakfast into her daily routine, hoping it would align with her body's natural morning rhythms. She found a few breakfast options that she was really excited to try out, aiming to promote regularity and digestive health from the start of her day.

Weekday: Overnight oats

25g jumbo oats, made with ~100ml milk (cows' or soya milk) and
    some 'live yogurt'
1 handful raspberries
1 tbs ground linseeds
1 tbs almond butter
1 large cup of coffee

Weekend: Avo-egg toast

2 slices favourite bread (wholemeal sourdough, rye or spelt bread,
    or soda bread)
2 eggs, fried in 1 tsp extra virgin olive oil
½ avocado, mashed with some lime juice and black pepper
½ tbs pumpkin seeds
½ tbs chia seeds
1 espresso

Result

During her follow-up visit, Joan successfully managed to get up and march into work a bit earlier, giving her a 15-minute window to have breakfast before logging on to her computer at nine o'clock. In fact, she fully embraced the 'morning routine' to help combat constipation: drinking a glass of water while getting ready for work, continuing to walk to work, enjoying a balanced breakfast (those options that included a selection of plant-based foods and wonderful fibres, healthy fats and live yogurt), and enjoying a cup of coffee after breakfast. She also incorporated the optimising toileting experience advice – more on this in Chapter 14 on toileting tricks. This routine set Joan up for significant success in her bowel movements, helping achieve a victory on the porcelain throne.

So it's not clear whether it was the breakfast itself, what she had for breakfast, that extra cup of coffee, or just taking the time to sit and encourage a bowel movement that led to Joan's constipation success. But you know what? It doesn't really matter! Having a morning routine that includes all these elements can be a real gamechanger for a lot of people dealing with constipation. Why not give it a try and see how it works for you?

•CHAPTER 13•
LIFESTYLE AND CONSTIPATION

Introduction

It's comforting to know that the main focus of managing constipation is on softening the stool, a simple yet effective strategy that works well for most people. When coupled with healthy eating, adequate fluid and regular meals, it's often the winning formula. However, if this has not been 100 per cent effective for you, it's time to continue to look beyond the basics and to consider other factors that can play a role in achieving happier gut days. This means adopting a holistic, panoramic view to understand and manage your condition fully.

In this view, there is a whole selection box of lifestyle factors that can play a role in overcoming constipation. Their effects can range from subtle to striking, and of course differ among individuals! From the impact of stress and anxiety to the effects of physical inactivity and sleeping habits, these connections might be unexpected, but they are indeed real and sometimes impactful. It's time to unravel their complexity, and most importantly to explore practical strategies to conquer their effects.

Mind over matter

But first, let's look at a range of key body systems to understand their potential role in the complex web of interconnections with the gut, and possibly constipation.

First, the enteric nervous system (ENS), your body's 'second brain', is crucial for regulating bowel motility. Any disturbances in how the ENS works could contribute to inconsistencies in bowel movements. Stress and gut issues such as constipation and IBS can alter ENS function by affecting its signalling and leading to changes in digestive function.

The ENS operates independently of the central nervous system (CNS) – the CNS is our first, or main, brain. However, it employs similar neurons and chemical messengers. In fact, that are up to 100 million nerve cells located within and operating entirely along the gastrointestinal tract, from the oesophagus to the internal anal sphincter. The ENS controls and regulates digestive functions within the gastrointestinal tract, helping it function properly.

These include those small segmenting movements that blend food with digestive enzymes and break it down further. The ENS also oversees peristalsis – the motions that push food through the oesophagus and the intestines, aiding in both mixing and moving the digestive contents. Moreover, the ENS is in charge of the MMC (see Chapter 12, page 170), another vital process that aids overall digestion.

There is also the vagus nerve, which is the bridge between the CNS and the ENS. It's one of the longest nerves in the body, extending from the brainstem down to the abdomen. Acting like a major communication line, the vagus nerve sends signals from the brain to the digestive organs and vice versa. This nerve plays a key role in controlling various digestive functions. For example, it helps control how quickly food moves through your stomach, the amount of stomach acid produced, and the relaxation of digestive muscles to make digestion work smoothly. It's like a messenger that carries instructions and feedback between the brain and the gut, ensuring that the digestive system works smoothly and efficiently. So, while the ENS can operate independently, the vagus nerve provides an important link that helps coordinate and fine-tune digestive processes in response to the body's needs and external factors. This is further facilitated by neurotransmitters, the body's chemical messengers, allowing the CNS and ENS to exchange information.

Next is the autonomic nervous system (ANS), which controls all the automatic functions of your body that you don't consciously think about, like your digestion, heartbeat and breathing. The ANS seesaws between two nervous systems: the sympathetic nervous system and the parasympathetic nervous system. These systems play a crucial role in how our body responds to stress and handles digestion. Let's take a closer look at them.

First, there is the sympathetic nervous system, which we affectionately call 'fight or flight' mode. When this system kicks into gear, it's all about preparing your body to deal with perceived threats. That means it redirects energy away from things like digestion because, well, survival comes first. So our gut motility can slow down, potentially worsening constipation. Chronic stress, which keeps the sympathetic nervous system on high alert, can be a culprit behind ongoing digestive issues such as constipation. Therefore, less of this 'fight or flight' mode is definitely a good thing.

On the flip side, there's the parasympathetic nervous system, aka 'rest and digest'. This system is your body's way of saying, 'Let's chill out and focus on digestion.' When the parasympathetic nervous system is active, digestion takes the centre stage, promoting a calm and relaxed state in your body. It's essential for efficient digestion and proper waste elimination. If you're dealing with constipation or IBS-C, getting more of this 'rest and digest' action can be a game changer.

In your day-to-day life, these nervous systems can quickly adapt to what's going on around you. Stress signals from your brain can divert blood flow away from your gut to vital organs like your heart and brain.

Conversely, when your digestive system isn't happy, it can send signals back to the brain, potentially leading to a change of mood and gut symptoms. While ongoing research is delving into this, an imbalance or prolonged activation of the sympathetic nervous system – often linked to long-term stress or anxiety – is thought to disrupt normal digestion.

To keep your digestion functioning at its best, we need to try to encourage our body's state of relaxation. When it's active, it increases production of stuff like saliva, digestive juices, enzymes and bile, all of which help proper breakdown and absorption of nutrients. Doing things that wake up your parasympathetic nervous system – like deep breathing, meditation and getting a good night's sleep – can give your digestion a boost and perhaps even ease constipation.

Then there's the HPA axis, or hypothalamic-pituitary-adrenal axis, which is a stress response command centre in your body. It's a network involving three parts: the hypothalamus (a part of your brain); the pituitary gland (a small gland at the base of your brain); and the adrenal glands (located on top of your kidneys). When you're stressed, this system also kicks into action: the hypothalamus sends a signal to the pituitary gland, which then signals the adrenal glands to release stress hormones, whose effects can slow down intestinal movement. Persistent stress, resulting in these higher hormone levels, can potentially make the intestinal walls more permeable (increasing leaky gut) and in some cases trigger inflammation, which could hinder digestive processes.

So, to sum it all up, the ENS (our gut's own brain) is the boss when it comes to running the show in our digestive system. It gets a helping hand from the ANS and CNS, our body's control centres. We can't forget things like stress hormones and the HPA axis, which are intertwined in all of this. Understanding these connections sheds light on the role of stress and how it can disrupt our digestive system, even though there are still many aspects that have yet to be fully understood. While it's perhaps an oversimplification to claim that reducing stress will directly lead to improved bowel regularity, it can't be overlooked.

One thing is certain: reducing stress can have a positive impact on our overall health, and that's something from which we could all benefit.

The stressed gut

In today's fast-paced world, chronic stress has become a common backdrop to our lives, influenced by factors such as demanding work environments, financial worries and the relentless pace of technology. Personal worries, health concerns, societal pressures and the pursuit of perfection all add to this stress. Being in a constant state of tension doesn't just affect our mental well-being; it can also have real consequences for our physical health, including the potential for constipation in those who are susceptible. It's important to remember that stress affects everyone differently. The way our bodies respond to stress can vary greatly from one person to another. For some, the impact on the digestive system may be quite noticeable, while for others it might be less so. The relationships between psychological aspects, stress and increased risk of constipation are discussed in Chapter 3.

The 'Stress–Constipation Connection' quiz

Welcome to the 'Stress–Constipation Connection' quiz!* This quick assessment is designed to explore the potential links between your stress levels, lifestyle habits and bowel health. Answer each question to the best of your ability.

1. How often do you find yourself in a constant rush, feeling on edge, stressed or anxious?

    A. Almost always
    B. Frequently
    C. Sometimes
    D. Rarely or never

*Please know that this quiz is for personal insight and does not replace professional medical advice.

2. Do you feel nervous or hesitant about using the bathroom for bowel movements when not at home?

    A. Yes, it's a major concern for me.
    B. Occasionally it can be a bit uncomfortable.
    C. Rarely. It's not a usual concern.
    D. No, I don't have any issue with it.

3. Can you recall an event or situation that led to a significant change in your bathroom habits?

    A. Yes, I can pinpoint an exact incident.
    B. There might have been an event, but I'm not certain.
    C. Not that I can recall.
    D. No, my habits have remained consistent.

4. How would you describe your 'stool expectations'? Do you feel they might be unrealistic or too rigid?

    A. Yes, I expect a certain outcome every time.
    B. I have some expectations, but I'm flexible.
    C. I don't have strong expectations.
    D. No expectations. I take it as it comes.

5. Do you notice a difference in the frequency of your bowel movements between weekends and weekdays?

    A. Yes, there's a noticeable difference.
    B. There might be a slight difference.
    C. I haven't noticed any pattern.
    D. No, it's consistent throughout the week.

6. Do you consciously set aside time to have a bowel movement without feeling rushed?

> A. No, I rarely give myself enough time.
> B. Sometimes, but it could be more.
> C. Often, but not always.
> D. Yes, I always make time for this.

7. Have you ever experienced a trauma or significant stressor that you feel has impacted your bowel habits?

> A. Yes, and it has had a lasting impact.
> B. Possibly, but I'm not entirely sure.
> C. Maybe a minor one.
> D. No, I haven't experienced trauma related to this.

The answers will be self-explanatory. Mostly A's indicates a high stress–constipation connection. More B's suggests moderate stress. Mostly C's indicates mild stress. Mostly D's means no stress to worry about!

What's constipation got to do with it?

As you can see, this connection between the brain and the gut holds significant intrigue. Therefore, any therapy that promotes relaxation and reduces excessive worrying or negative thinking can create a mindful environment that allows you to better understand your constipation situation.

There are various and usually feel-good ways to achieve relaxation and rejuvenation, which encourage the dominance of the parasympathetic nervous system – your body's inbuilt chill-out mode – and preserve the balance of the ANS. This will hopefully have a knock-on effect on your bowel. So check out these suggestions and set sail towards a more relaxed and smoother gut journey.

Suggestions to manage stress

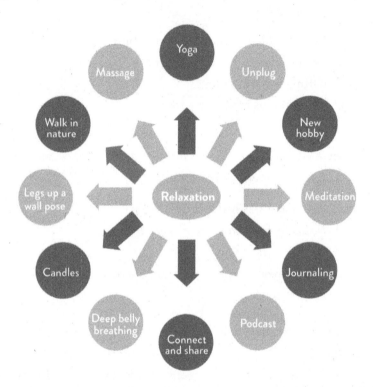

Even dedicating a mere five to ten minutes per day to any of these relaxation practices can have a beneficial impact on your stress levels, which may ultimately lead to a positive effect on your constipation.

'Legs up a wall' pose

The 'legs up a wall' pose is a soothing and accessible yoga posture that promotes deep relaxation and stress relief. This simple yet effective pose allows you to experience deep relaxation by gently elevating your legs against a wall! It is often used to calm the mind, reduce tension, and promote a sense of tranquillity. By practising this pose, you can easily release the stresses of the day and create a peaceful space for both your body and your mind to unwind.

Whether you're a seasoned yogi or new to yoga, the 'legs up a wall' pose offers a welcome escape from the demands of daily life, allowing you to fully embrace relaxation and rejuvenation.

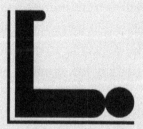

- Find a clear wall space. Choose a quiet area near a wall where you have enough room to lie down comfortably.

- Sit sideways. Begin by sitting on the floor with your side facing the wall.

- Move closer to the wall. Gently swing your legs up onto the wall while lying on your back. Your buttocks should be as close to the wall as possible.

- Adjust your position. Shift your body so that your legs are resting vertically against the wall and your back is flat on the ground. Your arms can be placed by your sides with your palms facing up.

- Relax and breathe. Close your eyes and take slow, deep breaths. Allow your body to relax in this pose.

- Stay for a few minutes. Hold the pose for 5 to 15 minutes, or as long as you're comfortable. You should start to feel more and more relaxed as time goes on.

- Come out of the pose. To exit the pose, bend your knees and roll onto one side. Rest for a moment before slowly getting up.

Remember to listen to your body and adjust the duration based on your comfort level. Don't let the simplicity fool you; the relaxation you'll achieve in this pose is worth trying.

Mind–body therapies

There are a range of specialist therapies that focus on the connection between the brain and the gut, such as cognitive behavioural therapy (CBT) and hypnosis – both of which can be specifically aimed at treating gut issues – as well as mindfulness-based stress reduction and yoga. There is also evidence that behavioural therapies are effective in addressing conditions like anxiety or stress. They can lead you towards a calmer, more controlled daily life, empowering you in your journey to better health.

Research suggests that therapies targeting the gut–brain connection are moderately to highly effective in managing gut symptoms of pain, bloating and distention, as well as helping constipation. If you're someone who suffers and who likes to weigh the odds, these findings might encourage you to consider these therapies. They're considered valuable complements to other treatments, such as dietary or medical approaches, in the management of gut symptoms.

Cognitive behavioural therapy

CBT is a really supportive kind of therapy that works on transforming unhelpful thought patterns. It's great at reducing stress and boosting your ability to cope well on your own. One of its super strengths is in tackling catastrophising – that unwanted habit of expecting the worst to happen. CBT guides you to gently observe and think about your thoughts and feelings. This can really help in easing psychological distress and dealing with pain. In IBS specifically, it has been shown that CBT decreases symptom severity, improves mental health and enhances quality of life, and that it's most effective when practised continuously or long term at home.

Mental flexibility

Any therapy that promotes relaxation and reduces excessive worrying or negative thinking can create a mindful environment that allows you to better understand your situation. One key component of this is 'mental flexibility', which is the ability of the mind to switch between thoughts or tasks and adapt to new situations. It's like mental yoga, enhancing flexibility and adaptability of the mind, allowing us to shift our perspectives, adapt to change, and approach challenges with a renewed outlook. Chronic stress can be influenced by a variety of factors, including rigid thinking patterns and difficulty adapting to change. Being mentally flexible means having the ability to adjust your thoughts and behaviour to changing conditions and stressors. This adaptability can help in managing stress more effectively, reducing its negative impact on the body, including the digestive system.

Constipation management often requires changes in daily habits – be they dietary changes, lifestyle modifications or, for some, increasing exercise. Someone with a mentally adaptable approach might find it easier to integrate these new routines into their lives, leading to more consistent and effective management of constipation. CBT is one way to enhance mental adaptability, and requires guidance from a trained healthcare professional. It can help you reshape or reframe your thought processes about bowel habits or assist you in successfully integrating new routines into your life, if you find them challenging. By rethinking any negative or stress-inducing perceptions about bowel movement or its treatment, you can adopt a more positive and calm approach to this essential bodily function.

Here are some real-life examples of how reframing can be used specifically for constipation management:

1. Situation: Tried to increase fibre in my diet and ended up feeling even worse.

    Original thought: 'Dietary changes never work for me. It's not worth it, I can't be bothered.'

    Reframed thought: 'Finding the right balance in my diet can take some trial and error. I think I should get support to help me do this properly.'

2. Situation: In a classroom or meeting where I can't simply get up and go to the restroom when the urge strikes.

   Original thought: 'I'm not able to leave, this is going to turn into a nightmare.'

   Reframed thought: 'I've managed situations like this before. For the good of my bowels, energy, mood and productivity, I need to discuss my needs with my boss to guarantee toilet trip flexibility.'

3. Situation: Hesitant to use the shared toilet at work because of potential smells and sounds.

   Original thought: 'This is going to be so embarrassing. I can't go because of the smell.'

   Reframed thought: 'Everyone uses these toilets and has their own moments. I deserve to feel comfortable. I can use air fresheners or white noise if I need to.'

4. Situation: Want to buy a dress for my friend's wedding but worried about looking bloated by the time dinner rolls around.

   Original thought: 'I can't wear anything nice because of my constipation.'

   Reframed thought: 'I have the right to feel gorgeous and choose a dress I adore. I'll select an outfit that not only looks stunning but also keeps me comfortable and self-assured all evening.'

5. Situation: At a friend's house and afraid to use their toilet in case it won't flush.

   Original thought: 'It will be mortifying if the toilet doesn't flush following my use.'

   Reframed thought: 'This can happen to anyone. If there's an issue, I can be honest and seek help. It's a human situation.'

By regularly practising the art of reframing your thoughts, you can transform your outlook from one filled with fear and avoidance to a more empowering and adaptable mindset. This technique doesn't dismiss the real challenges posed by constipation, but with practice this can become a powerful tool in one's arsenal for managing and coping with constipation. If you find this approach appealing, consider reaching out to a compassionate and experienced therapist who specialises in CBT. They can provide valuable support on your journey.

Gut-directed hypnotherapy

For those dealing with the difficulties of constipation and IBS-C, gut-directed hypnotherapy has emerged as a compelling and promising source of relief. Think of it as a therapeutic, gentle and feel-good approach to managing gut issues. Although the thoughts of hypnotherapy might sound a bit strange when you think of constipation, it's a legitimate therapy, firmly grounded in science and gaining recognition around the world. And just so you know, it's nothing like the hypnosis you see on stage or in entertainment – no purple cloaks or swinging watches should be involved. So if you do come across those, it might be a good idea to make a quick exit!

The technique harnesses the power of the mind to promote relaxation and harmony within the gut, potentially alleviating constipation and IBS-type symptoms. Whether you're seeking a drug-free solution or a complementary approach, gut-directed hypnotherapy holds great promise. This therapy not only helps in soothing the digestive process but can also calm the storm of stress and anxiety. and enhance overall quality of life. People who use it tend to find that relief is nearly always impressively maintained in the long run.

The exact ways in which hypnosis affects gut issues remain somewhat elusive. However, evidence from various studies indicates that the benefits of hypnosis might be down to two main factors: firstly, it can help regulate the functioning of the gut by reducing hypersensitivity;

and secondly, it can influence brain activity, particularly regions involving pain processing.

Gut-directed hypnotherapy employs a range of therapeutic techniques to promote relaxation and address digestive issues. At its core, this approach leverages progressive muscle relaxation, which helps individuals achieve a profound sense of calm. Deep breathing exercises are then integrated to relax the nervous system and reduce overall stress levels, facilitating the entry into 'an altered state of mind'. This altered mind state can be likened to a daydream or a state of flow, where one experiences deep relaxation while maintaining heightened awareness. You are not asleep. Neither are you fully awake! In this receptive state, individuals become open to messages and suggestions from their hypnotherapist, allowing for a more effective therapeutic experience.

Techniques then used to help exert the therapeutic effects include visualisation techniques, guided imagery and the use of metaphorical stories. For example, imagine you're introduced to a meandering river. Your therapist will guide you to visualise this river and explain that it's clogged in places, much like how your digestive system might be feeling. The therapist will then teach you how to unblock these obstacles in your mind, restoring the smooth flow in your digestive system, promoting regular and comfortable bowel movements. This simple yet powerful exercise can have a profound effect on people dealing with constipation and its associated symptoms.

Other techniques include ego strengthening (aimed at enhancing a person's self-esteem, resilience and sense of identity) and other mindfulness practices. Coping strategies can also be taught, giving individuals effective tools to handle stress and anxiety. Positive or reframing suggestions may also be offered to foster healthier bowel movements and habits.

Ultimately, this holistic approach tackles the psychological aspects intertwined with digestive issues, reducing stress, anxiety and negative thought patterns to support better gut function and overall well-being.

These techniques strive to reawaken the brain's built-in safety mechanisms, helping people recognise the difference between past triggers and the present moment. For those who experience stress-induced constipation and IBS, this approach can be highly effective.

Case study

Eve, a 24-year-old female, sought help for chronic constipation exacerbated by a history of IBS-C that worsened after experiencing COVID-19. Despite all the results of her medical investigations being 'normal', Eve endured persistent abdominal pain, bloating and incomplete bowel movements. She found some relief by adhering to a low FODMAP diet, and maintained a healthy and varied diet with adequate fluid intake. Eve enjoyed both running and yoga. However, she felt her recent transition to a demanding role as a trainee solicitor was related to worsening symptoms.

Treatment Plan: Gut-directed hypnotherapy

Eve completed six gut-directed hypnotherapy sessions over 12 weeks – which she found to be a thoroughly enjoyable experience. In these sessions, the focus was on creating a calm mental space, visualising smooth digestion, handling stress, strengthening positive habits and gaining self-control. Surprisingly, this therapy turned out to be the key element she had been seeking to find relief, and she started to really enjoy her improved bowel function and resolved gut symptoms. Her experience highlights the incredible influence of the mind–gut connection in dealing with gut issues, including constipation.

Mindfulness and meditation and the simple practice of slowing down breathing

More good news for those dealing with gut issues! Mindfulness isn't just a buzzword – it genuinely helps. Studies show that paying even a little more attention to the present moment can do wonders for our mental health, making us better at handling stress. While most of this research has been on people with IBS, the findings are pretty exciting. Imagine this: 42 per cent of people saw their IBS symptoms settle down with mindfulness. They also felt happier and less anxious. This is a natural and soothing way to take care of both your mind and body. So if you're navigating through the twists and turns of constipation, mindfulness might be a gentle, medication-free path worth exploring.

Mindfulness is about noticing your feelings and body sensations without any judgement – kind of like watching clouds pass in the sky. This amazing approach can make you feel better both mentally and physically, and it's really versatile – not just one thing. You can try it through meditation, when out for a walk or, of course, when you're tucking into your dinner. You can foster a sense of control and resilience in the face of constipation's challenges by nurturing your capacity to stay grounded in the present moment, engaging in enriching activities like reading, puzzles or acquiring new skills, and – again – reframing your inner dialogue.

Think of these mindfulness practices as a safe space for your mind, especially when constipation or gut symptoms are getting you down. They can gently guide your attention away from discomfort, sharpen your mental clarity, and offer a break from the cycle of worry and frustration. If you're open to trying them out, these practices could be the key to not only relieving physical discomfort but also giving your overall well-being a much needed lift.

Explore guided meditations or mindfulness apps to help you stay on track and deepen your practice. While Calm and Headspace are excellent choices, you can also explore additional options available in your app store.

Or how about trying out a breathing exercise? Deep belly breathing, also known as diaphragmatic breathing, is an excellent and simple way to relax. Engaging in slow, deep breathing exercises has been shown to promote relaxation, reduce stress reactions and even enhance something called 'vagal tone'. Vagal tone refers to the activity of the vagus nerve, that key part of your ANS that helps regulate various bodily functions. When you improve your vagal tone through deep breathing, it's like fine-tuning your body's internal mechanisms for relaxation management.

All you need to do is set aside a few minutes each day for this breathing practice. It helps to choose a specific time – maybe right after you wake up or before you go to bed – whatever works best for you. Find a cosy, quiet spot where you can relax without interruptions. Ready to get started? Here's your very simple guide to mastering an enjoyable breathing technique.

Diaphragmatic breathing technique

Sit or lie down	Sit or lie in a comfortable place. Close your eyes. If sitting, keep your shoulders, head and neck relaxed. If lying down, you can place a pillow under your knees for support.
Chest vs belly	Place one hand on your chest and one hand on your belly. The hand on your belly should do the moving. This will help you focus on the movement of your diaphragm as you breathe. The hand on your chest should not be moving.
Inhale	Inhale through your nose for about 4–6 seconds, feeling your belly expand or rise, pushing your hand out as far as it can go. Your chest should remain relatively still. You may feel slight tension during these initial inhalations.

Hold	Hold your breath for about 2 seconds.
Exhale	Exhale through pursed lips (like you're whistling), feeling the hand on your belly go inward. Use it as a guide to help push all the air out.
Repeat	Continue this pattern of deep, slow breaths for several minutes. Focus on the rise and fall of your belly.
Persevere!	Aim to engage in this breathing daily, for at least 8 weeks, to start to really notice the effects.

The secret to this breathing technique is to breathe nice and deeply from your diaphragm, not just taking short breaths from your chest. Imagine your breath reaching all the way down to your belly button – that's the sweet spot! This kind of deep breathing will relax your body (and gut). And here's a pro tip: try to make your exhale longer than your inhale, as that's like a magic button for your nervous system, helping it get into a super-relaxed state – the parasympathetic state.

Mindfulness-based stress reduction

Mindfulness-based stress reduction (MBSR) is a structured programme, usually an eight-week course, designed to help individuals reduce stress and improve their overall well-being through mindfulness practices. MBSR has been given the big thumbs up scientifically too, including in the gut world, for alleviating symptoms such as abdominal pain. Where there is a common element of heightened stress, mindfulness can step in, helping to dial down the tension and bring some much-needed peace to your day – again via the parasympathetic nervous system. The core idea is that individuals can reestablish a strong connection with their bodies and gain greater control over their physiological responses. So if you're looking for a gentle, natural way to feel better, this is another option that could be worth looking into.

Yoga

Yoga can also be something to explore for improving digestive health. Specific yoga poses, particularly twists and forward bends, could help promote movement in the gastrointestinal tract. Yoga not only enhances balance, strength and mobility but also fosters a mindful awareness of one's thoughts without judgement. Consistent yoga practice can enhance bowel movements and alleviate symptoms of constipation. Yoga's holistic approach, combining physical postures, breathing exercises and meditation, also contributes to stress reduction. In a study with older adults who hadn't tried yoga before, and who practised yoga three times a week for three months, participants reported notable improvements in sleep quality and constipation-related life quality. Those who practise yoga regularly have also reported improved sleep, as well as a decrease in depression and anxiety levels, alongside an improvement in overall quality of life. Win win!

Yoga can also be safe and effective for managing IBS. In many cases, its effectiveness has been found to match or even surpass the effectiveness of some pharmacological treatments for IBS. It also holds up well when compared with other non-medical interventions such as dietary modifications and moderate-intensity walking.

How to deal with stress

Stress management is a deeply personal journey, and we all have our own unique ways of finding relief. Whether it's taking a peaceful walk, sharing your thoughts with a close friend, simply doing nothing, or even exploring the mind–body or therapeutic techniques mentioned earlier, there's no universal remedy. What truly matters is that the stress-relief method you choose should authentically rejuvenate you, bringing a sense of peace and well-being to your life. The possibility of providing relief from constipation is an additional yet tangible bonus.

If you ever find yourself struggling to cope with overwhelming stress, it can be immensely beneficial to delve into the root causes and consider practical steps you can take to lighten the burden. Remember, it's completely okay to ask for help or take a step back when things feel overwhelming. Seeking support and exploring available resources can provide you with valuable tools and guidance on your journey to managing stress and improving your overall well-being.

Examples of support avenues

YouTube channels:
The School of Life; The Honest Guys

Websites:
Mindful.org; psychologicalsociety.ie; aware.ie; alustforlife.com

Apps:
Calm; Headspace; Smiling Mind; Stop Breathe & Think

Courses:
Google 'Mindfulness meditation' or 'mindfulness-based stress reduction' in your local area

Books:
The Happiness Trap (R. Harris); Introducing Mindfulness (T. Watt); Mindfulness for a Frantic World (M. Williams)

Managing stress

Spark joy
Art, walking in
nature, new hobby

Add activity
e.g. walk, cycle, swim

Connect and share
Tell people what's going
on, how you feel

Get mindful
Meditation, yoga,
breathing, prayer

Know when to get help
If reduced quality of
life, emotions take hold,
history of trauma

Conclusion

Overall, these practices could be helpful as part of the holistic management of constipation. They are brilliantly positioned to target your parasympathetic nervous system, outmanoeuvring the 'fight or flight' mode. So, for anyone navigating the slow road of constipation, adding CBT, gut-directed hypnotherapy, mindfulness, meditation, deep breathing and/or yoga to your routine might just be the secret ingredient you've been looking for. Keep an open mind – experiment with different methods to help you discover the perfect mix that fits just right for your unique journey.

Physical activity

Introduction

Getting active in your daily routine can potentially help kickstart your bowels into action by promoting intestinal movement. However, the full scoop on this connection between constipation and the bowel is still unfolding. Some evidence suggests that physical activities can enhance colonic motility for certain patients. But some studies have shown no clear link between exercise and transit time, which makes it all the more difficult to understand the real effects of exercise on constipation. Even if the impact on bowel movements is difficult to demonstrate, in one study involving middle-aged, non-active folk, although there wasn't a notable change in their weekly restroom rendezvous with exercise, there was a meaningful drop in their encounters with tough, incomplete or strained bowel movements.

Exercise has some interesting effects on our internal body clock, especially when it comes to how our colon contracts. As mentioned, changes in our daily circadian rhythms can have an impact on how our gut works and could be linked to constipation. When you do aerobic exercise, it might slow down the movements in your colon at first, but then it can actually help create a rhythmic pattern of pressure waves, which could in turn be helpful for moving stool along. Some experts feel that 'strengthening the core' can help improve bowel movements. Engaging in exercises may make your core muscles stronger and create more pressure in your belly. This extra pressure might help move things along in your digestive system. While there's still so much more to learn about how exercise affects constipation, it seems that a combination of aerobic and strength training exercises is going to be most helpful in speeding up the journey of waste through your large intestine.

Plus, staying active is the right thing to do, and many people find that exercise *can* alleviate constipation symptoms. It therefore remains part of the main advice when trying to get on top of this pain-in-the-ass condition.

Why engage in regular exercise?

Engaging in regular physical activity strengthens the heart, promotes optimal circulation and guards against cardiovascular troubles. From the strength of our muscles to the density of our bones, exercise ensures flexibility and reduces the risk of osteoporosis. Our lungs draw in air more efficiently. Adding in the regulation of blood sugar, a revved-up metabolism, enhanced energy levels, and enhanced immune defence, it's clear that the physical dividends are vast and to be welcomed.

Exercise doesn't just do wonders for our bodies. It's also a big win for our mental and emotional health. It's like a full package deal in boosting our overall well-being. It magically releases those beautiful mood-elevating endorphins and leads to improved and deeper sleep. While the evidence might still be in a debating zone as to how it directly impacts constipation, expert wisdom backs the view that physical activity is a valid ticket to smoother bowel movements.

How much is enough?

Engaging in a minimum of moderate-to-intense exercise, spanning 30 to 60 minutes, 5 days a week should do it.

Golden advice: Always sync your exercise routines with activities you love and that suit your personal health needs.

Sleep

Ensuring a good night's sleep is essential, acting as the backbone of overall health, including that of the digestive system. It's like reinforcing the foundation of a building, making sure everything operates smoothly and effectively. As we settle into bed and transition into sleep, it's not only our brains that enter a state of rest – our digestive system does too, in alignment with our circadian rhythm, as discussed already.

Unfortunately, many of us are sleep deprived. In fact, sleep disorders are a widespread global concern, and their prevalence is rising. The impact of sleep duration, whether too short or excessively long, has been extensively studied and linked to a reduced quality of life and adverse health outcomes. Despite this wealth of knowledge, scientifically the connection between sleep quality and gastrointestinal disorders including constipation has not been properly explored. However, people with constipation often report lower quality of sleep. This is particularly evident among full-time nurses working rotating shifts, who have shown a higher prevalence of constipation symptoms compared with their counterparts on regular daytime schedules. Additionally, research has observed links between sleep disorders, increased constipation, and levels of anxiety and depression.

Other fascinating patterns have emerged when trying to unravel the connections between sleep and constipation and IBS. Individuals who slept for unusually long periods and those who had notably short sleep durations were 61 per cent and 38 per cent more likely, respectively, to experience constipation. Around 33 per cent of those with IBS reported struggling with sleep disturbances. And when people with IBS had poor sleep quality on one night, they often reported increased symptoms the next morning – that is, they could predict gastrointestinal symptoms the following day if they had a poor night's kip.

For those with IBS, it's not just about the quantity of sleep, but also how restful that sleep is. When your sleep doesn't leave you feeling refreshed, it can make you more sensitive to pain and increase mental stress. This in turn can make the pain feel even worse. What's interesting is that there's a considerable overlap between IBS and chronic fatigue, with approximately 51 per cent of IBS patients also experiencing chronic fatigue. Dealing with both of these challenges can have a profound impact on one's ability to lead a normal life, as it can be extremely debilitating.

More important insights were unveiled when scientists made connections between our gut bacteria and our daily circadian rhythms. The metabolites generated by these gut microbes – for example, SCFAs – impact our internal body clock, our sleep patterns and even our physical make-up. When sleep is disrupted, it can throw off the balance of these microbes. Interestingly, some of these gut microbes, which become more active when you don't sleep well, can produce compounds that make you feel tired! Essentially, your sleep quality and the health of your gut are connected and can influence each other in a continuous cycle.

For now, the links between sleep, your gut, your circadian rhythm and constipation are still in their early research stages, with, we hope, ongoing exploration. However, as this link between the world of dreams and the rhythm of digestion has come to light, it does appear that our mental well-being and our gut microbes are intertwined in the whole story. Integrating this knowledge into your constipation treatment script could help improve the outcomes when seeking relief.

Tips to improve sleep hygiene

Sleep hygiene is a term used to describe having both a bedroom environment and daily routines that promote consistent, uninterrupted sleep. These are some helpful sleeping tips that you can try to implement into your day. If you struggle to get good-quality sleep, it is worth mentioning this to your GP.

10 sleep hygiene tips

Here are some tips that may help you improve your sleep hygiene.

- *Stick to a sleep–wake schedule* – Consistency is key. Go to bed and wake up at the same time every day, even on weekends, as it can regulate your body's clock.

- *Create a restful environment* – Make your bedroom a temple of rest – quiet, dark and cool, with comfortable bedding and minimal disturbances.

- *Limit exposure to screens* – Turn off electronic devices at least an hour before bedtime. The blue light they emit can interfere with your sleep cycle.

- *Reflect on your eating pattern* – Avoid heavy or large meals within a couple of hours of bedtime to prevent discomfort that might keep you up. Also, be wary of nicotine, caffeine and alcohol, which can disrupt sleep.

- *Get comfortable* – Wear comfortable night clothes and invest in a good-quality mattress and pillows to enhance your sleep.

- *Relaxation techniques* – Engage in calming activities before bed, like reading, taking a warm bath, meditation or deep breathing to signal to your body that it's time to wind down.

- *Exercise daily* – Regular physical activity can help you fall asleep faster and enjoy deeper sleep, but don't exercise too close to bedtime or you might be too energised to sleep.

- *Manage worries* – Try to resolve your worries or concerns before bedtime. Jot down what's on your mind and set it aside for tomorrow.

- *Get light exposure* – Natural light during the day helps maintain a healthy circadian rhythm. Try to get outside in natural sunlight for at least 30 minutes per day.

- *Nap smartly* – If you choose to nap during the day, limit it to 20–30 minutes. Late-day naps can interfere with nighttime sleep.

By fine-tuning these aspects of your daily routine, you can foster better sleep, which could well enhance your ability to improve gut health and manage constipation.

•CHAPTER 14•

TOILETING TRICKS

When we venture into the world of achieving smooth and effortless bowel movements, it becomes clear that we can't overlook the powerful influence of stress, the luxury of time or the significance of posture. Let's explore how these factors intersect and how to handle them to help coax your bowels into action and further shape the landscape of constipation management.

Too busy to go

Everybody needs to allow adequate time and privacy for bowel movements. This could be one of the most underrated constipation strategies out there. It's a certainty that the hustle and juggle of modern life can exert its influence on our digestive systems. But escaping its hectic pace – the daily grind – is a luxury reserved for the select few. Does any of this sound familiar – dividing your attention between the frenzied morning rush to leave the house, the crawl of the daily commute, the formidable mountain of paperwork and deadlines, not to mentions all those meetings to attend, before getting back on the road to attack the evening mayhem? If so, your bowels' needs might unintentionally be relegated to the shadows – stationary and stagnant. Your waste just settles in for an extended stay.

Is your daily visit to the loo a hurried affair, where you dash into a cubical, decide within 20 seconds that there's no urge for a bowel movement today, before rushing back to your desk to tackle the to-do list? Alternatively, are you among the diligent individuals who seldom have the chance to answer nature's call when it beckons, forcing you to suppress the urge? Perhaps you're the type who patiently waits for the elusive and clean unicorn public toilet or apprehensively avoids using outside-the-home toilets in general to shield yourself from potential noises or odours.

These situations represent missed opportunities, because it's essential to heed and address your bowels' desires. Your bowel, you see, is quite demanding when it comes to time – it likes to take things slowly and can be rather obstinate, because it is such a sensitive thing. Hence, it's crucial to try to create calm and provide the necessary time for it to function optimally. When we experience pressure or anxiety, or are just rushing and on the go all the time, and especially if we are toilet shy, our bowel can become uncooperative.

Plus, your bowel operates on its own schedule, often not in sync with your daily routine. From unfamiliar environments to changing time zones, it doesn't always easily adapt. Essentially it doesn't always appreciate the change of scenery. Nevertheless, it's crucial to bear in mind that having a bowel movement is a natural aspect of every individual's physical needs. It's a shared human experience and there's no need to feel embarrassed if you find you need 'to go'.

Poo anxiety

A wide range of individuals, from adults to children, often feel anxious about bowel movements. This condition, known as parcopresis or shy bowel, involves a struggle with using the bathroom in public places.

This anxiety might show up as avoiding bathrooms when others are present or hesitancy to travel because of public restroom use. Other anxieties intertwined with this can include fear of being far from a toilet, difficulty using the bathroom when necessary, and worry about cleanliness. The fear of judgement in public restrooms often leads people to rely solely on their home bathrooms, limiting their ability to leave home and potentially leading to unhealthy stool holding (refer to Chapter 3, page 47 for more details on why this isn't recommended).

Seeking therapy can be a beneficial approach to tackling parco-presis. A therapist can play a crucial role in uncovering the underlying causes of the fear associated with parcopresis and in offering strategies to manage it. Several therapeutic approaches have shown effective-ness, including gradual exposure therapy, which helps individuals become more accustomed to anxiety-inducing situations gradually, and CBT, which aids in altering thought patterns. Hypnotherapy can be used to address subconscious fears, while stress management tech-niques and relaxation training can help reduce overall anxiety levels. Implementing these therapeutic methods can be key in managing and alleviating the anxiety related to parcopresis, paving the way towards a more comfortable and confident experience.

Daily bowel movement routine

One of constipation management's primary rules is: Respond promptly to the urge to move your bowels. Try to not hold or put off a bowel movement. Sit on the loo and try to relax. When sitting on the toilet, it's important to avoid straining, as this can cause unnecessary stress on your body. Straining can lead to issues like haemorrhoids and anal fissures, and it can also put pressure on your pelvic floor muscles. To prevent these problems, maintain a relaxed posture and use all the tips here to allow bowel movements to occur naturally, without forcing them.

Firstly, try to move your bowels at the same time daily, ideally 15 to 45 minutes after breakfast (that meal you never skip!), as this is probably the most effective meal in helping to stimulate bowel motility. Beginning with this initial step towards regularity can be highly effective for so many people. Keep in mind that having a bowel movement every day isn't a strict necessity – remember bowel motions can vary from 3 to 21 per week. If you find yourself waiting for more than 10 minutes on the loo without results, there's no need to stress about it; just leave and go back to what you were doing. However, if you haven't had any movement for more than three days, then you're facing constipation and it might be time to take steps to address the issue.

If you are a constipation sufferer, it's important to grant your body the care and attention it deserves for this vital movement. Aim to allow up to 10 unhurried minutes for your bathroom break. Additionally, when it's in your control, consider creating a peaceful atmosphere in your bathroom, prioritising your privacy and comfort above all else.

Now, what if you're struggling to find even a spare five minutes for a morning bathroom break after breakfast? Well, here's a straightforward solution: wake up earlier! I know, that sounds like music to your ears, doesn't it? If it's feasible, even just try experimenting with an extended morning routine for a duration of three to four weeks to get a feel for its impact. Adjusting your sleep schedule might make it easier to rise and shine earlier and ensure there's ample time to tend to your needs in private. If you can't commit to that every day, focus on those less hectic days, like your precious weekends or days off. If your work situation doesn't exactly embrace bathroom freedom, consider dedicating 5 to 10 minutes for a toilet visit after a different meal, preferably when at home, which allows for a bit more flexibility.

Make the most of how you sit on the loo

In the quest for relief from constipation, sometimes the key lies in the angle. Our anatomy matters. The positioning of your legs can influence the alignment of your large intestine. When you squat rather than merely sit, you will naturally raise your knees above your hips, thereby relaxing your puborectalis muscle and straightening your rectum. This adjustment may make it easier for stools to pass out.

Toilet footstools are tools designed specifically for this purpose. However, you don't necessarily need a fancy stool – the simple act of raising your feet using a potty-training stool, stack of books or anything else stable can help achieve the desired position.

Anecdotally, some individuals have found footstools beneficial for facilitating more comfortable and effective defecation, although this hasn't been fully confirmed in clinical trials – another unpredictable finding all to do with the unpredictability of our unique bodies! Nevertheless, it's a simple and low-effort approach, so worth giving it a shot. Additionally, strengthening the pelvic muscles and anal sphincters can aid in facilitating smoother expulsion without unnecessary strain. Consider consulting a pelvic health physiotherapist for guidance on this.

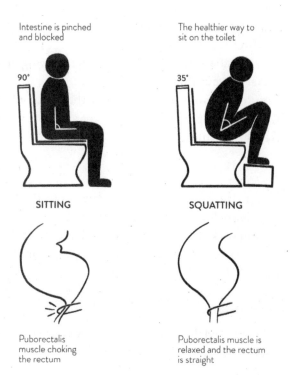

Intestine is pinched and blocked

The healthier way to sit on the toilet

90°

35°

SITTING

SQUATTING

Puborectalis muscle choking the rectum

Puborectalis muscle is relaxed and the rectum is straight

If you find yourself away from home and can't exactly whip a footstool from your backpack, don't worry. Simply altering your posture by changing positions can be quite helpful. Even if it's just a matter of engaging different muscles or finding a more comfortable position, it can help relax the abdominal and pelvic floor muscles to assist in making passage easier. Additionally, the rhythmic movement can provide a mental distraction and help you relax. You might discover how impactful a small change can be. Give it a try!

Toilet seat exercises

Here are four seated toilet stretches that can help promote relaxation and potentially aid in the process of defecation.

1. Deep belly breathing with forward lean
    - Sit upright with your feet flat on the ground.
    - Take a deep breath in, filling your diaphragm and expanding your belly (just like the instruction in Chapter 13, page 199).
    - As you exhale, lean forward slightly, bringing your chest closer to your thighs.
    - Ensure that your exhale is longer than your inhale, which will help you relax.
    - Repeat 10 times.

2. Pelvic tilts
    - Sit upright and place your hands on your thighs.
    - Gently rock your pelvis forwards and backwards.
    - As you rock forwards, your lower back will arch slightly; as you rock backwards, you'll tuck your tailbone under.
    - Repeat 10 times.

3. Knee-to-chest stretch
    - While seated, lift one knee towards your chest, using your hands to hold it in place gently.

- This can help stretch the glutes and lower back, and it may help to put gentle pressure on the intestines.
- Hold for a few breaths, then switch to the other leg.
- Repeat 10 times.

4. Ankle flexes

- Keep your feet flat on the ground.
- Lift the balls of your feet while keeping your heels on the ground to stretch the calf muscles.
- Then, point your toes downwards, lifting your heels. This stretches the front of your shins.
- Repeat 10 times.

Remember, these stretches are gentle movements. Remember too that no one is looking! Alternate between them to see what works for you. They're meant to help you relax and coax bowel movements, but they shouldn't be forced or cause any pain or injury. Always listen to your body and stop any movement if it feels uncomfortable. Seeking additional guidance from a pelvic health physiotherapist will help find the best approach for you.

Abdominal massage

When it comes to constipation relief, there's some intriguing evidence suggesting that abdominal massage might hold the key to quicker, more complete bowel movements. It's been touted as a cost-effective and gentle treatment. It has also been shown to reduce discomfort, bloating and straining, potentially offering a more satisfying experience and improved well-being, as well as reducing reliance on laxatives. However, as with many aspects of constipation-related research, larger and more rigorous trials are necessary to establish solid evidence regarding the clinical effectiveness of abdominal massage.

Abdominal massage is believed to stimulate peristalsis, the rhythmic muscle contractions responsible for moving food through the digestive system. It can create a ripple effect in the rectum, signalling to the body to have a bowel movement. This manual stimulation can help promote more regular and efficient bowel movements, possibly even making stools easier to pass. However, it's important to note that the exact mechanisms and effectiveness of abdominal massage may vary from person to person.

Abdominal massage has been a part of traditional practices in various cultures, where it is often combined with the use of traditional oils. The belief is that these oils enhance the therapeutic effects of the massage, and this practice has been used to help constipated patients.

It is possible to perform abdominal massage by oneself, but it's best to have an initial demonstration by a trained professional – for example, a pelvic health physio or nurse.

How to massage

Like all techniques, there are specific methods and precautions to ensure safety and efficacy. Here's a guide for a self-massage technique and the anatomical landmarks pivotal for a successful massage.

- Start by lying on your back. Slide a slim cushion under your knees or keep knees bent if that's more comfortable. This relaxed posture eases tension in the abdominal muscles, enabling a more effective massage.

- Take a few deep breaths to help your body relax and maximise the benefits of the massage.

- Quickly rub your hands together until they feel warm. Apply some massage oil if using.

- To start, place your hands on your belly, fingers pointing down-wards, palms making contact with the skin, and press down gently.

- Then move your hands to the lower back, massaging towards the stomach, as this is thought to activate the vagus nerve, signalling to the bowel to become active.

1. Then start massaging near the left side of your abdominal ribcage, stroking in clockwise circular motions down to the left hip bone. Repeat this 10 times.

2. Next, stroke from the right ribcage, underneath the ribcage to the left, and down to the left hip bone. Repeat this 10 times.

3. Lastly do 10 strokes from the right hip bone up to the right ribcage, across to the left ribcage, and down to the left hip bone. Repeat this 10 times.

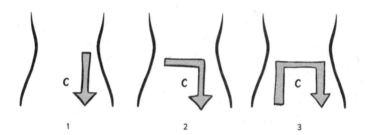

- Conclude with a vibration technique. Place your hands flat on your abdomen and gently shake them while they rest there. The movement should be small and rapid, resembling a subtle vibration. Keep your wrists relaxed and use your whole hand to create the vibration. This not only invigorates the nervous system but is also a nice tactic to ease muscle tension. Bonus: some people find it particularly handy in alleviating gas.

Massage tips

Using the flat part of your fingers and palm, make large, smooth circles in a clockwise motion. This follows the natural path of your intestines. However, if you feel bumps, you can begin lightly in the opposite direction to clear blockages, then proceed clockwise.

Apply gentle yet firm pressure as you massage. Your touch should be deep enough to stimulate the muscles and intestines underneath but never so hard that it causes pain. If at any point the massage feels painful or uncomfortable, stop immediately. It's always good to consult with a healthcare or massage professional if you're unsure about doing this yourself.

Precautions

It's crucial to know when *not* to attempt self-massage. If you have any of the following conditions, refrain from abdominal massage, or consult with a specialist:

- post-abdominal surgery
- active infections, cancer or chemotherapy in the pelvic area
- abdominal aneurysm
- rectus diastasis (the separation of the two long vertical abdominal muscles)
- active diverticular disease
- suspected blockages
- appendicitis
- other concerning health conditions, especially in the abdominal area.

Morning constipation routine

1. *Hydrate.* Begin by sipping a glass of water that you've strategically placed on your bedside locker the night before. While this might not have a scientific explanation, it's a practice that many find beneficial in hydrating the body and possibly aiding in bowel function. Hydration can set a positive tone for your day.

2. *Activate your muscles.* Incorporate abdominal massage, gentle stretching or movement into your routine. If you find it challenging to fit them into your schedule, consider doing these exercises before bedtime as an alternative.

3. *Eat.* Prioritise a balanced breakfast to kickstart your day. Opt for a meal rich in fibre (include some of the foods that have been shown to work), adding some healthy fat, and perhaps including some fermented milk or yogurt. A breakfast like this can provide essential nutrients and support digestive health, setting the scene for optimising bowel movements and working with your body's natural rhythms.

4. *Have a hot drink.* As part of your morning routine, consider enjoying a caffeinated beverage in descending order of preference: a mug of coffee, a mug of decaffeinated coffee, a mug of tea, a green or herbal tea.

5. *Take time.* Then find that window (15 to 45 minutes after breakfast) to take a moment for yourself on the loo. Sit down on the toilet and relax. Stretch, reposition and breeeeathe. Never hold your breath! The diaphragmatic breathing technique can be useful here. Also, do your best not to strain. If you're feeling particularly anxious or nervous, you could also listen to calming music or repeat a positive mantra.

6. *Observe.* As you continue to breathe slowly, steadily and deeply, pay close attention to several physical and mental signals that indicate your body is embracing relaxation. Feel your shoulders gradually releasing tension, lowering down and relaxing back. Observe your abdominal and pelvic muscles softening. Take notice of your facial muscles as well, particularly around your eyes and jaw. Are they becoming less tense? A relaxed facial expression is often a strong indicator that your body is at ease. Physical sensations may differ for everyone, but try to recognise them, as they help signal that your body is preparing for a natural release. If racing thoughts start to quieten down, and your mind feels more at ease, these are other positive signs that your body is responding to relaxation techniques.

7. *Be patient.* Your bowel is more likely to cooperate when it feels secure and at ease.

Case study

Assessment

In Beatrice's daily life, where she relished working from the comfort of her home, an unexpected challenge emerged when she found herself back in the office environment. Her well-established morning routine, which included staying hydrated with water, enjoying a fibre-rich breakfast, and savouring her coffee, had long kept her digestive system running smoothly. It was a well-rehearsed performance that left her feeling in control.

However, the office presented her with a new obstacle – the toilet situation. It was a single, cramped cubicle with a finicky lock and questionable flushing capabilities. In response, she made a conscious choice to avoid using the office restroom, even when her body signalled the need. She believed this was the safer option given the circumstances. As days turned into weeks, Beatrice began to experience the consequences of her decision. Bloating and gas became her unwelcome companions. The rhythm was off!

Plan

Upon realising the importance of the 'call to stool', Beatrice was determined to regain her comfort and regular bowel rhythm.

Unable to find a suitable alternative toilet at work, she had to improvise. She made it a point to get up 30 minutes earlier, use the toilet at home after her 'morning routine', ensuring she addressed her body's needs before heading to work. Additionally, she employed some of the toileting tricks such as deep belly breathing and positioning her knees above her hips to entice those care-free bowel movements.

Outcome

Beatrice's commitment to her bowels' needs paid off. By prioritising toilet time post-breakfast at home and using effective toileting techniques, her bowel movements became regular again.

Beatrice's journey serves as a testament to the power of adaptation and consistency, and to the importance of honouring our body's signals. It's a story that anyone who has fought with constipation can undoubtedly relate to.

Approaches for defecation dyssynergia

Biofeedback

Another approach some have found helpful is biofeedback, which can be used to target the defecation dyssynergia we covered in Chapter 3 (page 36) – that inability to coordinate the muscles of the pelvic floor and abdominal wall during bowel movements, leading to difficulty in passing stool. This condition can manifest as straining, incomplete evacuations, and often a sense of frustration and discomfort. The good news is, once the muscle issue is treated, gut speed and function can return to normal.

Pelvic health physiotherapy offers a range of interventions designed to address the root causes of this condition and provide relief, and in the next few paragraphs we will explore this world and the various evidence-based interventions it offers to improve the lives of those affected by defecation dyssynergia.

When dietary changes, lifestyle tweaks and even laxatives don't quite do the trick to ease your constipation, it's time to consider alternative approaches that target the functioning of the anorectal (rear end) region. Keep in mind that while specialised pelvic floor therapy might not be readily available everywhere, the good news is that it's becoming more recognised and accessible. So there's hope for finding the help you need.

If you are showing signs of issues with rectal emptying based on your assessments, biofeedback may be a treatment option for you. Not only may it help with irregular or hard bowel movements, but it has also been shown to reduce abdominal discomfort and bloating. One nice thing about biofeedback is that it doesn't come with any side effects.

In fact, there's a study that suggests it might even work better than laxatives over a six-month period. So it's definitely worth considering if you're dealing with this issue.

How it works

Biofeedback is like a supportive teacher for your body. It's a technique that helps you take control of things that your body usually does automatically, like freely moving your bowels. The goal is to teach you how to relax your pelvic floor muscles when you need to have a bowel movement and to pay better attention to how full your rectum feels. This awareness helps you know when to push just right to make things go smoothly.

Biofeedback methods come in different forms. Some practitioners will use sensors, balloons or hands-on techniques to help you feel and understand what your muscles are up to. The hands-on approach – where a trained therapist guides you through muscle relaxation and control – is common, but really each practitioner is likely to have their own way of doing things. And for those who might not feel sensations in their rectum very well, biofeedback also helps you get better at recognising and responding to those feelings, allowing you to tune into bowel movement signals again.

If all of this sounds a bit intrusive, don't worry. You'll be in capable hands with a skilled healthcare provider. Experiencing a bit of apprehension when considering the idea of someone assessing your private inner muscles is entirely normal. It's also a highly personal and intimate aspect of your health that you may not have discussed openly before.

Just a friendly reminder: these experts are here to support you and have seen it all before. Take a deep breath, try to be open and honest about your concerns, and trust in their expertise. Your comfort and well-being are their top priorities.

It's important to note that studies have demonstrated short-term success rates of around 70 per cent and long-term benefits for approximately half of the patients who have undergone biofeedback therapy, which is really quite impressive. The effectiveness of this treatment depends on the expertise of the therapist and the dedication of the patient. While ongoing research is underway, it's worth highlighting that biofeedback is widely recognised as an effective approach for managing constipation associated with persistent muscle issues.

Psychological support

If biofeedback is not effective, a psychologist may get involved. Pelvic health physiotherapy focuses on addressing the physical aspects of conditions like pelvic floor dysfunction and dyssynergia. However, it's important to recognise that many individuals with these conditions may also have underlying emotional triggers. Factors like trauma, childhood toileting issues and chronic stress can contribute to these pelvic health challenges. This is where psychologists come into the picture.

Psychologists conduct thorough psychological assessments to identify any underlying psychological conditions or stressors that may be contributing to constipation. They employ evidence-based behavioural interventions, including CBT, to assist patients in modifying thought patterns and behaviours that could worsen their condition. Additionally, psychologists may provide biofeedback therapy to assist individuals in managing stress-related physiological responses. This can help the person gain control over physiological functions such as pelvic muscle relaxation, which is particularly relevant in cases of pelvic floor dysfunctions. Managing stress is another crucial aspect of a psychologist's work, as stress and anxiety can significantly impact bowel function. Psychologists help individuals explore the mind–body connection and offer supportive counselling to address the emotional challenges often associated with constipation.

In summary, the combined approach of physiotherapy and psychological support recognises that pelvic health is not just about muscles and mechanics; it's about the whole person. By addressing both the physical and emotional aspects, this approach offers a comprehensive solution for those seeking relief from pelvic floor issues. It's a personalised journey towards better pelvic health and overall well-being.

Holistic approach

Taking a holistic approach to managing defecation dyssynergia can make a real difference, and therapies like biofeedback become even more exciting when combined with other strategies. This can cover a range of helpful practices, including tips on the right way to use the toilet, finding the best position for bowel movements, and incorporating effective breathing techniques. Plus, it includes a tailored dietary plan to keep your stool soft and manageable. But that's not all. Having a supportive therapist, especially if stress is a major factor in your condition, and consulting with a doctor for a review of your medication, if necessary, can truly improve your chances of finding relief and achieving overall well-being if you're dealing with these issues. So, you've got a winning hand of options to explore.

•CHAPTER 15•
THE BIOTICS

Probiotics

The term probiotic, arising from Greek, translates as 'for life.' In the early 20th century, Élie Metchnikoff, a renowned Russian zoologist and a pioneer in immunology, introduced the revolutionary idea that consuming fermented milk products could inhibit the growth of harmful bacteria in the gut. This insight paved the way for the concept of modifying the gut microbiome with beneficial bacteria and a significant advancement in the understanding and management of gut issues.

The term 'probiotic' was initially introduced in 1954, and its definition has been rewritten in various ways since then. The most current and precise definition is that probiotics are live microorganisms that when taken in appropriate amounts provide health benefits to the person consuming them. This means that when you take probiotics, they should have a noticeable effect; otherwise, there's no point in taking them!

Probiotics are in the spotlight these days, and are being researched and marketed as affordable and safe options for helping to manage various chronic conditions, from diabetes to depression, alongside gut disorders like constipation and IBS. These minuscule organisms can include beneficial bacteria, as well as specific types of yeasts and fungi. You can find them in many different forms, including capsules, liquids, powders and chewable tablets. They are also added to a diverse range of products, with yogurt and other fermented milks being among the most popular choices for delivering probiotics.

The most intriguing thing about probiotics is that they are highly specific to their strains. When it comes to bacteria families, only a few members might have those proven probiotic abilities and have the desired beneficial effects. Take *Lactobacillus acidophilus*, for example. One type could work wonders for a particular health issue, but a different variation of the same species might not do anything. The key is to try to discover the right one for the right situation.

While it's true that trendy fermented foods like kimchi, kombucha, kefir and yogurt are often praised for their potential probiotic benefits, not all of them can be labelled as true 'probiotics'. The probiotic label is earned when scientific research confirms their health-boosting properties – that is, through clinical trials. So, when you're looking for probiotic products, it's a good idea to seek those with proven benefits for specific issues, like promoting more regular bowel movements. If they work for you, they can be a valuable addition to your health routine. And if not, don't worry—there are plenty of other options to explore.

Probiotic names

When selecting probiotics, it's helpful to grasp the different classification levels: genus, species and strain. These categories assist in recognising and categorising bacteria according to their genetic and biological traits. Understanding these classifications can be a bit confusing at first, but it's essential for making informed choices about probiotics. Let's use *Bifidobacterium lactis* BB-12 as an example.

Genus. Think of the genus as a big family that includes different species that share some similarities. For instance, when we talk about the probiotic bacteria Bifidobacterium, 'Bifidobacterium' is like the family name in the world of bacteria. It's the first part of their scientific name.

Species. Think of species as the smaller, more specific groups within the genus. They have their own unique characteristics. For example, in the name *Bifidobacterium lactis*, 'lactis' is like the first name of these bacteria, and it helps us tell them apart from other species in the Bifidobacterium genus. It's the second part of their scientific name.

Strain: Strains are like the unique individuals within a species. They have tiny genetic differences that can make them behave differently or have different effects. For example, think of *Bifidobacterium lactis* BB-12 as a particular member of the *Bifidobacterium lactis* family. These strains often have names made up of letters and numbers that come after the species name, giving each one its distinct identity. It's the final part of their scientific name.

Choosing a probiotic to relieve constipation and associated symptoms

Choosing the right probiotic for constipation relief has its own challenges. Unlike some other digestive conditions like IBS, where probiotics have shown promise in relieving symptoms like pain and bloating, the evidence supporting their role in managing constipation with a view to increasing nice soft and bulky stools is not as strong. So, it's important to keep in mind that while probiotics might help with constipation, there's still a question mark around their effectiveness in this specific area.

As mentioned, probiotics are highly strain specific, and their impact on individual bodies can vary significantly. Consider the example of two individuals, Anna and Emily, both dealing with constipation. Anna finds a probiotic supplement online that brings her substantial relief within a week. Emily, inspired by Anna's success, tries the same supplement but doesn't experience similar benefits. This scenario mirrors how people respond differently to medications for other conditions, just as one person's migraine might respond to an anti-inflammatory drug while another requires a serotonin-receptor agonist. In the same way, the probiotic strain that worked wonders for Anna's constipation might be well suited to her unique gut composition, whereas Emily's gut might respond better to a different strain or a different approach altogether.

That's because our bodies' existing conditions and the condition of our gut microbiota can significantly influence how probiotics perform. Some strains may thrive more effectively when there's not already a substantial population of similar bacteria in the gut. On the flip side, probiotics may sometimes compete with or suppress existing gut bacteria, leading to a complex balance of potential advantages and disadvantages. Different probiotic strains can also respond differently depending on what's in your diet, and individual variations in digestion and metabolism will finish it off with one more layer of complexity.

Current research is keenly focused on trying to pinpoint who can benefit most from probiotics. For example, some dietary elements may boost the activity and growth of probiotic strains. Combining high-fibre foods with probiotics, like consuming high-fibre rye bread alongside probiotic yogurt, has shown potential in managing constipation. This combo resulted in increased daily bowel movements and softer stools. Interestingly, while rye bread alone could sometimes lead to minor gastrointestinal issues, adding yogurt seemed to alleviate these side effects, highlighting the possible synergistic effects of combining fibre and probiotics – more on synergy in a moment! This research sheds light on how dietary fibre, along with probiotics, interacts with bowel activity.

It's worth knowing that probiotics only remain in your gut temporarily. Instead of taking up permanent residence in our gut, probiotics usually make a temporary stop, making changes as they pass through. So to reap the benefits of probiotics, you need to take them consistently, every day, without interruption. They exert their effects through several key actions, including helping to combat harmful pathogens by taking up space in the gut; influencing gut microbiota composition; reinforcing the gut lining; enhancing immune function; and supporting the gut and the brain – to complement and support your own in-house microbes.

In a nutshell, probiotics have the potential to help with constipation, but their effectiveness depends on a variety of personal factors and what your own gut microbes are up to at that time. So, when it comes to probiotics, it's all about finding what works best for you and your unique gut ecosystem.

How to take a probiotic

1. Start by picking the perfect strain: Probiotic strains have different functions. Go for a probiotic that matches your particular health goals, whether it's addressing constipation, related gut issues or stress.

2. For optimal results, take your probiotic supplement at the same time each day. Some strains work best when taken on an empty stomach, typically in the morning, while others are more effective with meals. Check the label for specific instructions.

3. Regularity in taking your probiotic is crucial. Set a routine to incorporate the supplement into your daily regimen. Remember, the benefits of probiotics are seen with continuous use.

4. Store your probiotics as recommended, often in a cool, dry place. Some may require refrigeration. Always check the expiry date to ensure you're consuming a potent product.

5. Enhance the effectiveness of probiotics by maintaining a balanced diet rich in fibre, fruits and vegetables. This not only helps manage

your overall constipation status, but it should also create a friendly environment for probiotics to flourish in your gut.

6. Take the probiotic daily for an initial period of 8 to 12 weeks. Thereafter it's crucial to assess its impact. If there's no improvement, it's time to stop its use and explore either an alternative probiotic strain or other approaches for symptom relief.

By following these guidelines, you can navigate the world of probiotics with confidence and decide whether to incorporate them into your management plan or look in another direction.

Evidence supports trialling a probiotic, as the benefits outweigh the risks.*

Choose a probiotic that has shown benefits in constipation or associated symptoms, and take the suggested dose.

Trial × 2–3 months and evaluate success.

If not effective, try another brand or stop taking them.

* Individuals with severe health conditions or weakened immunity should consult a healthcare provider before using probiotics.

Why consider probiotics for constipation?

The possible benefits of adding a probiotic for constipation range from quicker movement through the gut to improved consistency of bowel movements. The exact science behind how probiotics aid constipation is still under investigation. In one in-depth analysis, probiotic intake reduced gut transit time by an average of just under 14 hours and increased bowel movements by 1 per week. They could also accelerate the speed at which food moved through the digestive system by about 12 hours.

Additionally, some strains have shown an effect on increasing bowel movement frequency, improving stool consistency, and reducing bloating. However, while these benefits have been observed, there's still a clear need for more targeted and consistent research to help figure out which probiotics are most effective for constipation relief, the ideal dosage, the optimal duration for consumption and which people they will best suit.

Strains that have scientific backing to help manage constipation

Understanding which strains have been studied and shown to provide constipation relief is, as outlined, a crucial step in finding a suitable solution for this digestive challenge. Below, strains that have shown promise in scientific studies for relieving constipation are highlighted. To determine which one may work best for you, it's advisable to consult with your doctor or dietitian and opt for reputable brands.

	B. lactis DN-173 010
	Bifidobacterium lactis BB-12
	Bifidobacterium lactis HN019
	L. reuteri DSM 17938
	Lactobacillus plantarum LP01 and *Bifidobacterium breve* BR03

Despite there being an appetite for clear-cut evidence to validate their use for constipation, at present the use of probiotics is likely best regarded as experimental. Although these specific microbial strains have emerged as potential allies in the quest for relief, you need to set realistic expectations. The effectiveness of probiotics is not predictable. Don't expect them to fully resolve your constipation.

Strains that have scientific backing to help manage IBS-constipation

The use of probiotics in treating IBS has gained more acceptance and positive feedback from people taking them, particularly for their role in helping alleviate related symptoms such as pain, bloating and gas. They can also help stress-related symptoms and improve well-being. If you're contending with constipation and IBS-type symptoms, the strains listed below may offer some relief.

	Lactobacillus acidophilus DDS-1
	Bifidobacterium longum 35642 ± Bifidobacterium longum 1714
	Lactobacillus plantarum 299v
	Bifidobacterium bifidum MIMBb75
	B. breve, B. longum, B. infantis, L. acidophilus, L. plantarum, L. casei, and L. delbrueckii subsp. Bulgaricus, Streptococcus salivarius subsp. Thermophilus

Safety concern

Probiotics are considered as safe agents for alleviating constipation and IBS symptoms in adults. They are typically well tolerated, with rare reports of adverse reactions identified in the trials published to date. However, safety is paramount, especially for vulnerable groups, including those who are immunocompromised or who are critically ill. As with any supplement, it's advisable to consult with your health-care team and obtain tailored recommendations before making any decisions.

The future? Next-generation probiotics

Considering all the things that are needed for a probiotic to be effective, it's not always as straightforward as matching a strain to a condition to quickly resolve symptoms. Some people will respond, but others won't. However, when evidence-based strains are chosen, the chances of an impact on symptoms are significantly increased.

The landscape of probiotics is likely to evolve significantly in the next decade. 'Next-generation probiotics' are at the forefront of this evolution, marking a significant leap beyond traditional strains like Lactobacillus and Bifidobacterium. These advanced probiotics introduce a variety of new, selectively chosen bacterial strains, currently under intensive research for their distinct health benefits.

What distinguishes these next-generation probiotics is their precision-targeted approach, which holds potential for revolutionising the treatment of conditions such as IBS and constipation. They may offer specific advantages – such as anti-inflammatory properties, direct improvement of gut motility or correction of gut bacterial imbalances – to pave the way for more customised treatments. Let's hope this move towards personalised probiotic therapy provides more efficient and individualised solutions for constipation and broader gut health issues, to minimise the need for so much guesswork.

Prebiotics

Prebiotics are the part of foods we eat – mostly plant-based foods – that positively alter the composition or activity of our gut bacteria. This should then lead to health benefits. They act as nourishment for the beneficial microbes in our gut. When gut microbes eat (that is, ferment) prebiotics, they produce those delightful short-chain fatty acids (SCFAs) we talked about earlier.

Prebiotics have been found to enhance bowel regularity, with an increase in stool frequency by about one additional bowel movement per week. They also help improve stool consistency, making bowel movements smoother. However, how they affect our gut is complex and not always easy to predict. Different prebiotics can encourage the growth of different types of microbes, and our gut's environment can change how these bacteria grow and interact, meaning the impact can vary from person to person.

The good news is that prebiotics are naturally present in a wide array of foods, including garlic, onions, leeks, dates, green bananas, oats, barley, linseeds, mango, chickpeas and lentils. It's thought to be more advantageous to firstly consume a wide range of plant-based foods to increase your prebiotic intake before considering supplements, as the foods offer more varied sources of prebiotics, along with a broad spectrum of essential nutrients such as vitamins, minerals and various beneficial plant compounds, including antioxidants. These nutrients work synergistically in the body, offering health benefits that supplements alone might not provide. Additionally, probiotics are dietary fibre, which you will hopefully agree is a friend of constipation.

You can also find prebiotics like fructo-oligosaccharides (FOS) and galacto-oligosaccharides (GOS) in supplement form. Remember inulin, one of the fibre supplements we mentioned earlier? Well, it's a type of FOS and is therefore a prebiotic supplement. If you're interested in trying it, you can refer back to Chapter 8, page 118 for more information on how to take it. In some constipation trials, people who took FOS or combined FOS with other sources of fibre saw an increase in the number of bowel movements and improved intestinal transit per week. And GOS, acting as an α-galactosidase, also increased stool frequency and had a positive impact on gut microbes, which is exactly what prebiotics are supposed to do! It's an exciting area of research.

However, it's important to know that many of the specific products with proven benefits from these trials are either still in the research stages or are not yet available for purchase. But this landscape is likely to change as more data are collected and benefits are further confirmed. In the meantime, to ensure that both you and your gut bacteria benefit — and consequently, your bowels — the best approach is to include a wide variety of plant-based foods in your diet first, supplements second.

Synbiotics

Now, imagine combining probiotics and prebiotics together. That's where synbiotics come in. The idea is that by giving our gut both beneficial bacteria (probiotics) and the food they love (prebiotics), they enhance each other's effects. Synbiotics aim to enhance the beneficial effects of both probiotics and prebiotics by working in synergy.

The health benefits of a synbiotic will largely depend on the specific pairing of its probiotic and prebiotic components. Research generally indicates that synbiotics encourage the growth of beneficial gut bacteria, particularly Lactobacilli and Bifidobacteria. Given the countless potential combinations, synbiotics hold great promise, and there are some emerging positive findings with specific combos helping enhance bowel regularity in patients with constipation.

However, one of the hurdles is that the outcomes are not always as expected. Although not common, in some instances, instead of enhancing the benefits by merging a probiotic with a prebiotic, the effect might actually be lessened. This inconsistency arises from the complex interactions within the gut microbiota, the strain-specific effects, the dose and formulation and, once again, the fact that each person's gut environment is unique! Additionally, the possibility of a placebo effect is a possibility. Synbiotics that combine FOS or GOS with probiotics may be the most effective combinations, but once again more research on this is needed to help establish more solid and reliable recommendations for synbiotics, especially in the case of constipation relief.

Postbiotics

Now let's talk about the lesser known postbiotics. These include a variety of substances produced by microorganisms as they go about their metabolic activities. These substances can encompass a diverse range of compounds, including vitamins, enzymes and SCFAs. They can be defined as inactive or non-living microorganisms or their components that confer health benefits. Ultimately, postbiotics cannot replicate, and as they are not alive, they cannot cause infections. This may offer advantages over probiotics, especially for immunocompromised individuals or in different product formats, and they could be more effective in maintaining microbiome diversity.

Postbiotics can sometimes be found in fermented foods like kefir, kimchi, sauerkraut, tempeh and yogurt, as they often contain a considerable number of inactive microbial cells, especially after long storage or processing methods like pasteurisation (such as commercial miso) or baking (like in sourdough bread). Certain foods are believed to be particularly effective at generating beneficial by-products in the gut. These include foods rich in prebiotic fibres and some yogurts, as they can encourage the production of helpful gut metabolites.

There are no studies to date to say postbiotics will help manage constipation. But if you're interested in maximising your chances of incorporating postbiotics into your diet, it's sensible to focus on consuming a diet rich in prebiotic fibre, fermented foods and polyphenols –

that is, eat more whole grains, vegetables, fruits, legumes and a variety of nuts and seeds! Some common examples of polyphenols include quercetin in apples and onions, resveratrol in red wine and grapes, and catechin in green tea. Other sources include berries, cocoa, turmeric, soybeans and extra virgin olive oil.

Current clinical trials focusing on postbiotics are still in progress, and while the initial findings are promising, it's important to note that it's still early days. We need more data! Just be aware that postbiotics sold in supplement form are not recommended at this time because of a lack of evidence.

Conclusion

The ongoing debate surrounding the effectiveness of various 'biotics' in treating constipation can be quite the head-scratcher. While many trials investigating treatments like probiotics, prebiotics and synbiotics for chronic constipation have reported positive outcomes with minimal side effects, the results are often a mixed bag because of numerous influencing factors. This makes it challenging to determine their true impact and provide good advice.

When it comes to selecting a probiotic, remember that a targeted approach is crucial. Avoid the *grab-any-probiotic-off-the-shelf* strategy or getting swayed by anecdotal recommendations from heavily marketed brands. Probiotic strains that sound similar can have hugely different effects on your gut. The key is to choose a strain with strong clinical evidence supporting its benefits. Keep in mind that what works wonders for someone else may not be your magic solution. And maintain realistic expectations about the results you can expect.

•CHAPTER 16•
LAXATIVES

What's the deal with laxatives?

Anyone who has felt the wrath of constipation knows just how challenging it can be. Sometimes, making dietary and lifestyle adjustments may not be sufficient to ensure everything moves smoothly. Let's take a look at the numbers. In Europe, a significant 68 per cent have tried using laxatives. The not-so-great news? Only 28 per cent of them found the relief they were looking for, no matter which kind of laxative they experimented with.

Finding the right laxative is again all about tailoring a solution to your specific needs, so seeking personalised advice to discover the laxative that suits you best is a sensible move. It helps to know your unique type of constipation – whether that's normal transit, slow transit, disordered defecation or IBS-C. It's also a sage move to know when to start and when to stop using laxatives, and to be aware of their potential side effects.

Always consult with your doctor or pharmacist for personalised advice, and remember, detailed information about each product is usually available inside the product's packaging.

Laxative choices

When it comes to laxatives, you've got quite the menu to choose from. They come in different varieties, including bulk-forming, osmotic or stimulant laxatives, softeners, suppositories, enemas and even some newer prokinetic options that promote intestinal motility in severe cases of constipation. Each type of laxative has its own special way of helping with constipation. The ones you'll often see first on the list are the trusty bulk-forming and osmotic laxatives. They're reliable and easy on the wallet, and they usually don't cause too many side effects.

Bulk-forming laxatives

We've touched on this topic before – ring any bells? That's right, our friend fibre is back in the limelight again. Bulk laxatives are usually derived from natural ingredients such as psyllium husks, and others are synthetic wonders with tongue-twisting names like methylcellulose and polycarbophil. Bulk-forming laxatives, aka specific types of fibre, take a gentle and unhurried approach to help you achieve regular and comfortable bowel movements. These types of fibre resist getting absorbed in the small intestine and are pretty resilient against the bacteria in the large intestine (if you remember from Chapter 8, they are soluble, viscous and low-fermentable fibres). This means they can hold on to water, which in turn increases the volume of stool in your bowels, resulting in softer and smoother movements.

It's important to know that if someone has a severe stool blockage or is at risk of faecal impaction – when a hard mass of stool becomes stuck in the rectum or lower colon and is difficult to pass naturally –

they should avoid using bulk-forming laxatives. This underscores a relevant point: even though they might seem 'natural' and therefore harmless, it's wise to have a chat with your GP before considering them. Your health comes first.

Psyllium husks take the crown as the leader of bulk-forming laxatives for boosting stool frequency; the others, unfortunately, not so much. Take a little journey back to Chapter 8, page 114, where you'll find a complete and interesting psyllium husks overview waiting for you.

Osmotic laxatives

Osmotic laxatives, as their name implies, induce an 'osmotic' effect, which means they draw certain molecules (ones that don't get absorbed) into your colon. This friendly invitation causes more water to be secreted by the intestinal lining and held in the large intestine. Your stool gets a boost in moisture and volume, making the journey through your intestines smoother and, hopefully, leading to a poo that's softer and much easier to pass. Some familiar faces in the osmotic laxative family are polyethylene glycol (PEG), lactulose, sorbitol, mannitol and magnesium salts.

Have you heard of or ever had a colonoscopy? If so, you might remember the interesting 'prep' phase – those unforgettable trips to the loo after drinking that special cleansing mixture. That potion, often a PEG solution mixed with electrolytes, is a perfect example of an osmotic agent doing its thing. When taken in such high volumes, it cleans out the bowels with remarkable speed.

Polyethylene glycols

Obviously, these osmotic laxatives are not prescribed in such large quantities for daily use! However, one of the most prescribed osmotic laxatives is PEG, which is also known as macrogol. It turns out it seems to be a top osmotic performer – making bowel movements more regular, improving the texture of stools and limiting tummy discomfort, as well as being particularly helpful for those with IBS-C. This laxative will need to be prescribed by your GP.

Lactulose

Lactulose is another osmotic laxative, which is basically a fermentable sugar and acts like a prebiotic (food for your gut microbes). The outcome is softer and bulkier stools. The general agreement is that lactulose has its perks for easing constipation for quite a few people. But the aftermath of the party with the microbes may lead to a build-up of gas in about 1 in 5 people. This could result in side effects such as abdominal pain, bloating, and in some cases diarrhoea, especially in those with IBS-related constipation. This laxative can be got over the counter. You should take as recommended by your healthcare provider or as per packet instructions.

Magnesium

Magnesium is an essential mineral that plays many vital roles in our bodies, including keeping our muscles and nerves strong and our bones healthy. But guess what? It has another cool trick up its sleeve – some forms can also act as osmotic laxatives. Common forms of magnesium supplements for constipation include magnesium citrate, magnesium oxide and magnesium hydroxide (also known as Milk of Magnesia). Among these, magnesium oxide often comes out on top, as it's minimally absorbed and so seen as typically safe.

However, there are a few cautions to keep in mind when taking magnesium supplements. Firstly, they are seen more as an effective quick-fix remedy for occasional constipation rather than for continual use. This is because consistent intake can lead to an electrolyte imbalance, notably elevated magnesium levels in the blood or hypermagnesaemia – a side effect that's not on your wish list.

This leads us to the second point. While high levels of magnesium are a potential risk with excessive intake of magnesium supplements for everyone, it's more commonly a concern for individuals with impaired kidney function. The kidneys typically regulate magnesium levels effectively, but when they are not functioning properly, the risk of accumulating too much magnesium increases. It's wise to get your blood magnesium levels checked, especially if you're dealing with chronic kidney issues or if you're on a high dose of magnesium oxide. And lastly, excessive doses can also result in diarrhoea – *not* what you're trying to achieve!

Dosing of magnesium

For adults, there's no standardised dose – once again, it's an individual thing! The smartest move is to start small and increase slowly. The effective doses can vary quite a bit, ranging from 250mg to 1,000mg daily, which just goes to show how differently different people can respond to it. Some might find relief with a small increase, while others may require more. It's important not to exceed 1,000mg per day. And don't forget to accompany your supplement with a good ol' glass of water to keep yourself well hydrated. It's best taken before bed.

So before rushing out to purchase magnesium supplements, make sure you (1) know which form you need; (2) decide the dose and know how much is too much; (3) use as a temporary constipation solution; (4) discuss having your magnesium levels tested; and (5) discuss all of these points with your doctor!

Lubricants and stool softeners

Alongside the popular bulk and osmotic options, some may turn to lubricants and stool softeners too. These are known for being gentle and well tolerated by most people. Lubricants are mostly non-toxic mineral oils such as paraffin oil. Their main gig is to stop water and salts from being absorbed, which can be a real help if you're occasionally backed up. But it's good to keep in mind a couple of things. If you use them a lot, they might mess with how your body takes in vitamins that need fat to work. And be careful how you take them, as there's a small chance of breathing them into your lungs if they're not taken correctly. Because of this, they are recommended for short-term rather than long-term use.

Stool softeners, with docusate being a prime example, boost the water and lipid content in stools, ensuring they remain soft and less challenging to pass. Unlike some remedies, they don't help trigger bowel movements; they merely soften the stool. Both lubricants and stool softeners are available over the counter. Just make sure to follow the instructions on the label to get the best results. While they might not be everyone's go-to choice, they're still recognised options when it comes to easing constipation.

Stimulant laxatives

Stimulant laxatives play a role in managing constipation by directly stimulating the activity of the intestines. Common examples of stimulant laxatives include senna, bisacodyl and aloe vera. They work by remaining dormant in the small intestine and then springing into action in the colon, encouraging both intestinal movements and secretion. These effects are achieved either by mildly irritating the intestinal lining or by directly activating the intestine's nerve networks.

Stimulant laxatives are typically deployed as rescue remedies, particularly for individuals who've not had a bowel movement for a while – for example, no bowel movement for three days or longer. They're also the backup plan when other types such as bulk-forming or osmotic laxatives don't quite do the trick. They can be very useful when you're in a tight spot and you need to get out of it.

Senna and bisacodyl are available over the counter. A heads-up, however – some people might feel a bit of stomach discomfort or even get diarrhoea after taking them. So, while they can get the job done, it's good to use them wisely. Always take as advised by a healthcare professional and read the label instructions before taking them. This way, you'll know exactly how to use them safely and effectively.

Healthcare providers might raise concerns about the 'potential dangers' of using stimulant laxatives, which may make people hesitant to use them. So in case you need to hear this, there's no convincing evidence to support the idea that using them as a laxative harms your colon. Some people may need to take them for extended periods. Your doctor can tailor the doses to fit your needs perfectly, making sure you get just the right amount for you. As with all laxatives, the same counsel holds true – take laxatives correctly and use them under the supervision of a medical expert.

Aloe vera, another stimulant laxative, is available in gel, juice and capsules, but may be best taken in liquid form for constipation. Aloe vera is a potential go-to remedy for those dealing with constipation and IBS-C, as it can offer symptom relief with no notable side effects. As a general guideline, start with a small dose, such as 50 to 100mls (about 2 to 4 tbs) per day. This can be adjusted up or down based on your body's response and tolerance.

However, although rare, aloe vera has been observed to be a culprit behind serious liver damage. For constipation, therefore, take advice from your healthcare professional, choose a trusted brand, and in the usual fashion, start with a smaller dose to see how your body reacts to aloe vera. Don't exceed the recommended maximum dose. Remember, more isn't always better, especially when it comes to herbal supplements!

Suppositories and enemas

When constipation gets bad, a trusty suppository can step in for fast relief. It's smoothly inserted into the rectum, where it works like a charm to draw in water, making stools soft and easing the way for a comfortable bowel movement.

Then there's an enema, the Ferrari of laxative treatments. When you receive it, a lubricated tube is gently inserted into your bum, usually a few inches, to ensure that the liquid can flow freely into the colon, where it helps soften up the stools and kickstart those lazy intestinal muscles. Both can offer constipation relief but are generally seen as short-term solutions for when faecal impaction is present – meaning stools are difficult to pass.

Prokinetic laxatives

Intestinal secretagogues

The latest entrants in the arena of constipation relief, known as intestinal secretagogues, are making a grab as additional effective laxative choices. These clever substances work by encouraging your intestines to release more fluids and boost the secretion of salts such as chlorides. This helps get things moving. Linaclotide and plecanatide are two options that have got the thumbs up for being both effective and safe. Side effects are pretty rare. Your doctor will be the one to give the green light and to write you a prescription.

Serotonin 5-HT4 receptor agonists

Expanding on our earlier discussion in Chapter 4 (see page 62), where we unveiled serotonin's crucial role in promoting movement in the gut, scientists have now crafted medications known as serotonin receptor agonists that tap into this pathway. One example of these agonists, prucalopride, works by boosting the activity of nerve cells in the intestines, which has been demonstrated to lead to better digestion. These types of laxatives are usually only prescribed after other laxatives and interventions have been explored. It might be worth having a chat about prucalopride with your doctor.

Laxative ladder*

	Type	Examples	Time needed to work
1st choice	Bulk laxatives** Stool softeners	Psyllium, methylcellulose	12–24 hours
		Docusate	24–48 hours
2nd choice	Osmotic laxatives	Lactulose	24–72 hours
		Polyethylene glycols (PEG)	24–48 hours
		Magnesium, e.g. oxide, citrate	30 minutes– 6 hours
3rd choice	Stimulant laxatives	Bisacodyl Senna	6–12 hours
Rescue therapy	Lubricants	Mineral oil	About 8 hours
	Suppository	Glycerin	15-60 minutes
	Enema	Microlax	5-15 minutes
When other laxative options fail	Intestinal secretagogues	Linacoltide Plecanatide	12–48 hours
	Serotonin 5-HT4 receptor agonists	Prucalopride	Varies from days to weeks

* Always get advice from your GP, gastroenterologist or pharmacist regarding the most suitable laxative for you, and take as advised

** Avoid if there is a risk of faecal impaction

Laxatives summary

Wrapping it up, think of laxatives as potential game-changers for those caught in the vice grips of persistent constipation. And some people will need to take something to move their bowels, just like someone who needs to take medication for their diabetes or blood pressure. Before diving into the laxative promised land, it's essential to tread carefully, however. You will need to have the necessary candid conversation with your doctor and ensure the choice aligns with your unique situation. Also, just because a laxative is available over the counter doesn't mean it's free from side effects or safe for continuous use! And don't give up on any of the other helpful strategies when using laxatives: continue your high-fibre diet and ensure you're hydrated, remain mindful of lifestyle factors, and optimise toileting rituals.

When taking laxatives, remember to not be too hasty. Some laxatives can sometimes take up to three days to fully kick in. Try not to rush the process; instead, give your body the time it needs to respond to the treatment. What's important is finding a rhythm that works for you and sticking to it for the best results. The role of laxatives is to ease symptoms while you work on restoring your body's natural digestive rhythm. Once you've regained regularity, you might discover that you can eventually reduce or even completely eliminate the need for laxatives in the long run.

If laxatives don't do the trick, it's like your body is whispering a secret clue. It's time to play detective and dig a little deeper. Consider it a nudge to chat again with your GP and get a referral to a consultant gastroenterologist, a pelvic health physiotherapist and/or a dietitian if you haven't already chatted with these experts. Keep it in mind that there's a whole world of other strategies out there, not just laxatives.

Laxative anxiety

'Laxative anxiety' is a term that describes the real and common concerns people have about using laxatives. It's usually driven by the fear of dependence, yet recent findings challenge this belief. It was recently shown that even after a year of use, the body did not get too used to the stimulant laxative bisacodyl. In other words, people didn't need to increase the dose first prescribed by their doctor. In real life, the danger with laxatives is usually observed if someone goes overboard and uses too many for a long time. As with anything, moderation is key!

If, however, you've ever had an overwhelming experience with laxatives, whether you're caught in a situation with or without a toilet in sight, it can leave a significant imprint on your psyche. Mentally, the incessant worry around achieving bowel regularity and potential dependency can also become a significant stressor. This might lead to a vicious cycle: anxiety exacerbates constipation symptoms, which in turn lead to increased laxative use, fuelling further anxiety.

Tackling laxative anxiety starts with arming yourself with information. Having read about how laxatives work, does it demystify their use? A candid conversation with your doctor can also alleviate fears and provide medical reassurance. Make sure to follow the recommended usage to prevent any unwanted effects – slow and low, everyone, slow and low! If anxiety looms large, don't hesitate to reach out for professional support. And remember, reshaping gut health doesn't happen overnight, so arm yourself with patience and keep a steady pace on your journey to more effortless departures. All in all, the information we have tells us that laxatives are a safe and effective way to relieve constipation.

Non-pharmacological approaches to manage constipation

Colonic irrigation versus transanal irrigation

Colonic irrigation, often known simply as a colonic, is a procedure where somewhere between 20 and 40 litres of water is infused into the colon, purportedly to remove waste and toxins. However, it's worth noting that your colon is self-cleaning, so why do you need a colonic? Well, you don't, primarily because colonics can actually disrupt the natural workings and inhabitants of your colon. You don't want to do that – they are too precious.

Colonics performed incorrectly can also harm the delicate tissues in your rectum and colon, sometimes leading to serious issues like when a hole forms in the bowel. The importance of sterility cannot be overstated – using an unsterile device can heighten the risk of infection. Frequent colonic use may disrupt your body's electrolyte balance and could result in nausea, abdominal pain and bloating. Additionally, apart from stripping away beneficial bacteria, there's the risk of introducing unfamiliar microbes – yikes!

In contrast, transanal irrigation (TAI) can be introduced as a medically supervised alternative to colonics, specifically designed for managing severe constipation and related conditions. Unlike colonics, TAI is a targeted medical procedure with a clear therapeutic goal. It's a controlled and safe method, typically involving the introduction of a smaller amount of water (about 500ml) into the bowel. It is self-administered under medical guidance.

Surgery

Living with chronic constipation can be so very challenging, enormously affecting your everyday life. However, considering surgery is not routine, is an absolute last resort, and is a really big decision. It's only considered when all other options have been exhausted. Before thinking about surgery, your medical team will thoroughly assess all risks, benefits and possible outcomes. Your health and well-being are always going to be the primary concern, and so your doctor or surgeon would only suggest surgery after a detailed examination of all factors and having had an in-depth conversation with you.

What does the future hold?

Faecal microbial transplant

Imagine taking a thriving gut community of microbes from a healthy individual and transplanting it into yours. That, in a nutshell, is a faecal microbial transplant (FMT). Here's how it works. Stool from a donor who has been deemed super-healthy is collected and processed to ensure only the beneficial microbes remain. This precious microbial load is then introduced into a patient's gut.

Why would someone consider this? Our gut is a bustling metropolis of bacteria, and a balanced community ensures optimal digestion and overall health (flick back to Chapter 2 for more on this). Should your body's intricate pathways become clogged, as in persistent constipation, the concept is akin to inviting outside exemplary inhabitants into the mix to smooth out the internal gridlock.

FMT has shown remarkable results for some stubborn infections. Preliminary constipation studies with FMT proved it to be more effective in improving bowel movement frequency, stool consistency and colonic transit times in both constipation and IBS-C. However, it was not without side effects. Although there are indications of its effectiveness, the available data on this subject is only short term, and a complete understanding of how it affects the gut bacteria is yet to be defined. As you can see, there are many uncertainties, but it's an exciting time with researchers exploring some intriguing possibilities.

If you find centres offering FMT, be careful. They are not a recommended treatment for constipation or IBS. There have also been some unexpected consequences reported that are as fascinating as they are unusual. For example, there's the story of a patient who, after undergoing FMT, and who previously disliked marmite, found themselves suddenly craving marmite, as the doner was a marmite lover. Another notable case involved significant weight changes: a lean individual received a transplant from an overweight donor and experienced unexpected weight gain, despite maintaining their usual diet and exercise routine. Mood alterations and anecdotal reports of individuals feeling as though their 'gut instincts' or decision-making processes changed following the procedure are other curious side effects.

Oh, one last thing: on social media a new trend is emerging in which people can be instructed to make a 'here's one I made at home' version of FMT and self-administer these stool samples. This can be from partners, family members or friends. This practice completely overlooks the potential health risks and complications that can arise from hidden health issues in the donors. Don't do it!

The vibrating capsule

In the quest for groundbreaking methods to tackle constipation treatment, a novel drug-free remedy has emerged – a vibrating capsule. Yes, that's right – a capsule that you swallow to help you achieve those sought-after and highly prized complete, spontaneous bowel movements.

The capsules are roughly an inch in size, embedded with a tiny battery and crafted to start vibrating when they reach the colon. The idea is that you take them twice a day, five days a week. They are pre-programmed to initiate two-hour 'vibration sessions', stimulating the colon for three seconds, followed by 16 seconds of inactivity. Scientists feel the gut–brain axis is also involved, and that over time the brain may learn to replicate these effects independently, without the need for the capsules. Once they have served their purpose, the body naturally expels the capsules. People who have taken these vibrating capsules observed double the number of effortless and satisfying bowel motions, reduced straining, improved stool consistency and overall well-being.

Are you wondering if you feel the good vibrations? Well, yes, but only 11 per cent mentioned a faint vibrating feeling within their abdomen, which they did not seem to mind. This groundbreaking device has garnered the green light from the US Food and Drug Administration (FDA), opening the door for its potential global adoption. Europe is waiting!

It's crucial to emphasise that discussing constipation with your healthcare provider should never be a source of embarrassment. If you've been dealing with ongoing constipation without relief, it's important to reach out to a medical professional. They have the expertise to address these issues and provide tailored solutions that align with your unique needs.

PUTTING IT ALL TOGETHER

Congratulations! You've reached the final chapter of our journey to better understand and manage constipation. Along the way, we explored all the relevant aspects of this common digestive issue, and we acknowledged that the struggle is real. But remember, where there's struggle, there's also the potential for solutions, and in the case of constipation there's a whole range of valuable, safe and proven strategies to address it. Now it's time to bring it all together into a comprehensive plan for optimising your digestive health.

Core strategies for constipation relief

1. Increase fibre and fluid intake.

- Gradually increasing your fibre intake is the cornerstone of managing constipation. Fibre adds bulk to your stool and promotes regular bowel movements.

- Begin by selecting the recommended fibre-rich foods that align with your taste preferences and gradually introduce them into your diet.

- Remember that a slow and steady approach is often the most effective way to increase fibre without discomfort.

2. Embrace regular meals.

    - Maintaining a consistent meal schedule supports healthy digestion. Aim to include a breakfast and two other main meals each day. Eat at fairly regular intervals to keep your digestive system in sync.

    - Avoid skipping meals, as well as irregular eating patterns, grazing and nighttime eating.

3. Use deliberate relaxation strategies.

    - Deep breathing exercises, meditation, yoga and spending time in nature can help you unwind and reduce stress levels.

    - Stress can have a profound impact on your gut health. Incorporate stress management techniques into your daily routine to minimise its effects.

    - If this is not helpful, consider gut-directed hypnotherapy, CBT or counselling with a trained and suitable healthcare professional.

4. Use the toileting optimising tricks.

    - Pay close attention to your body's signals and respond promptly when you feel the urge to have a bowel movement.

    - When it's time to use the restroom, create a relaxing environment. Take deep breaths, sit comfortably and allow yourself to fully relax during the process. Don't strain.

Peripheral strategies for constipation relief

1. Chew your food.

   - Chewing your food thoroughly aids in digestion. Take your time to savour each bite, breaking down food particles for easier absorption.

2. Include other gut-healthy foods.

   - Healthy fats – found in avocados, nuts, seeds, and extra virgin olive oil – can contribute to smoother digestion. Incorporate these into your diet.

   - Fermented foods like yogurt, kefir, sauerkraut and kimchi can support gut health. Consider adding these to your diet for their potential benefits.

3. Trial a probiotic.

   - Some individuals find relief from constipation by taking probiotic supplements. Use evidence-based products and discuss your options with your healthcare provider to determine if it's suitable for you.

4. Prioritise quality sleep.

   - Adequate sleep is crucial for overall health and digestion. Establish healthy sleep hygiene habits to ensure restful nights.

5. Engage in physical activity.

   - Regular exercise can help stimulate bowel movements and promote a healthy digestive system. Incorporate physical activity into your routine.

6. Consider bowel massage.

   - Gentle abdominal massages may alleviate constipation symptoms for some individuals. Explore this technique with caution and consider professional guidance.

When core strategies aren't enough

If you've diligently followed the core strategies and continue to experience constipation, it may be time to explore further options:

1. Seek a medical assessment.

    • Consulting a healthcare provider for a thorough evaluation is crucial. They can identify any underlying medical conditions contributing to your constipation.

2. Explore pelvic floor assessment.

    • In cases where pelvic floor dysfunction is suspected, a pelvic floor assessment can provide valuable insights and guide treatment. Signs that this is needed include sensations of straining and incomplete evacuation. In such cases, fibre and laxatives may not be as effective.

    • Biofeedback therapy can help train your pelvic muscles for more effective bowel movements. It's a valuable option for certain individuals.

3. Consider a trial of laxatives.

    • Your healthcare provider may recommend a trial of laxatives to provide relief from both short-term or long-term constipation. Always use them under professional guidance.

The importance of monitoring

Throughout your constipation management journey, keeping a detailed journal, from time to time, of your symptoms, dietary changes and improvements can be an empowering and supportive tool – like the template used in Chapter 3, which can be downloaded online. This can also serve as a valuable resource when discussing your condition with healthcare professionals.

Putting it all together

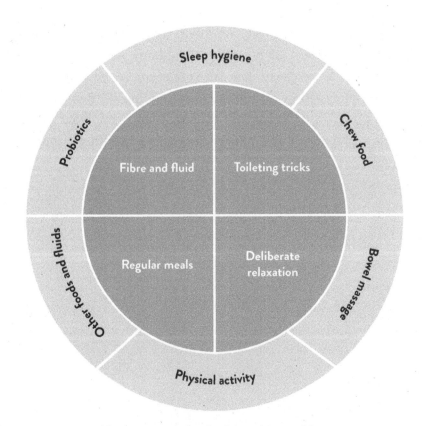

If core strategies don't work, consider:
1. Laxatives
2. Biofeedback
3. Psychological support

Your ideal healthcare support team

Your healthcare providers, especially those with expertise in constipation and disorders related to the gut–brain interaction, are invaluable allies on your journey to digestive wellness. Don't hesitate to seek their guidance and expertise as you work towards improved digestive health.

In conclusion

Managing constipation is a personal journey that can require patience and dedication, and a holistic approach. By combining core and peripheral strategies, seeking professional guidance when necessary, and monitoring your progress, you can regain control of your digestive health and enjoy a more comfortable and fulfilling life. Remember, you have the power to take charge of your well-being, and your digestive health is a vital part of that journey. Here's to a healthier, happier gut, and you!

•ACKNOWLEDGEMENTS•

Writing this book was made possible by the incredible support and expertise of some very special colleagues, family and friends, who mean the world to me, and for whom I am truly grateful.

Firstly, thank you to the very talented and professional team at Gill Books, especially Sarah, Aoibheann and Mia, for guiding me through this publishing journey.

Thank you to Dr O'Donovan, Consultant Gastroenterologist at Blackrock Clinic, whose insights and thoughtful feedback on the laxative chapter were not only needed but also provided invaluable wisdom for the entire book. I am equally grateful to Eimear Murphy, specialist pelvic health physiotherapist, also at Blackrock Clinic, whose necessary and practical guidance steered the comprehensive investigation into all things pelvic floor related throughout this book. Additionally, a sincere thank you to Niamh Forster, senior dietitian, for your crucial assistance with my research endeavours.

I am also grateful for the encouragement from all my other colleagues at Blackrock Clinic, especially my fellow dietitians, whose insights and engaging conversations offered a much-needed outlet for reflection. You were more influential than you may realise.

To all the Cooneys, especially my parents, whose steadfast support and encouragement helped to keep me grounded on several occasions. And to all my friends who cheered me on and helped me believe that this book would actually see completion.

And last but certainly not least, the biggest thank you is for Lilah and Edith, who have been impressively patient as I spent countless hours in front of my laptop. Thank you for not hiding it from me. This book is for you.

INDEX